# STRESS
## and Strategies
## for Lifestyle
## Management

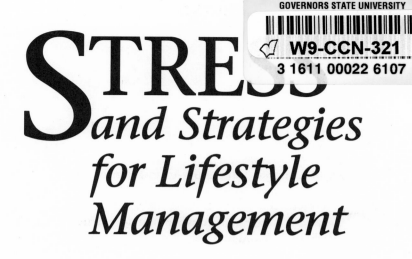

Kenneth B. Matheny, Ph. D.
*Counseling and Psychological Services*
*Georgia State University*

Richard J. Riordan, Ph. D.
*Counseling and Psychological Services*
*Georgia State University*

1992

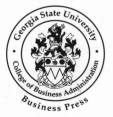

<blockquote>
Georgia State University Business Press
College of Business Administration
Atlanta, Georgia
</blockquote>

**The Library of Congress Cataloging-in-Publication Data**

Matheny, Kenneth B.
   Stress — and strategies for lifestyle management / Kenneth B.
Matheny, Richard J. Riordan.
      p. cm.
   Includes bibliographical references and index.
   ISBN 0-88406-250-3
   1. Stress management.   I. Riordan, Richard, J.   AII. Title.
RA785.M38 1992                                      92-7078
155/9'042-dc20

Georgia State University Business Press
University Plaza
Atlanta, Georgia 30303-3093

© 1992 Georgia State University

96 95 94 93 92        5 4 3 2 1

Georgia State University, a unit of the University System of Georgia,
is an equal educational opportunity institution and an equal
opportunity/affirmative action employer.

Printed in the United States of America.

Cover design by Patton H. McGinley, Jr.

To our wives, Mary Matheny and Barbara Riordan, and the combined seventy years of marriage. These partners have taught us much about the co-management of family stress.

And to our children—Carolyn, Ron, Janice, and Kurt Matheny, and Steve and Chris Riordan—who have been the joys of our lives.

# CONTENTS

## PART II
### Strategies for Changing Stressful Lifestyles

# PREFACE

Few topics have garnered as much attention in so brief a period as has stress. It has become the official bogeyman of our day. It is blamed for everything from headaches to heart attacks. It is said to create emotional anguish, to endanger one's health, and to shorten one's life. Much stress is caused by poorly managed lifestyles, and changes in one's thoughts and behaviors often are necessary to cope more adequately with stress. Much is known about stress, stressors, and stress symptoms, but much *mis*information exists as well. In this volume we seek to share the facts about stress and the process of change, and in doing so we empower readers to cope more effectively with the pressures of life.

We are creatures of habit. While most habits serve us well, some contribute greatly to the stress of daily living. To cope successfully it is sometimes necessary to change stress-inducing habits and conditioning. Change is never easy, but some strategies work better than others. In this volume we identify effective strategies for producing change in self and others. Confusion regarding *how* to change kills the nerve of moral endeavor. Clear maps and strategies for change create hope, and hope creates the energy necessary for change. Knowing *how* replaces helplessness with a sense of control and mastery; and many believe that this sense of control is the most effective buffer against stress.

While we experience a buoyant sense of freedom and power when we take charge of our lives, we feel constricted and stressed when life seems out of control. There is an inborn need within all of us to run our own lives, to create our own destinies. Henley expressed this need when he wrote "I am the master of my fate; I am the captain of my soul," and the writer of the popular song expressed it equally as well when he exuberantly declared "I did it *my* way!"

This drive for self-determination is spreading across the planet Earth. Entire societies are caught up in revolutions for self-control. Throughout the world people are clamoring for the right to manage their own affairs. Workers, students, family members, all of us function best and are healthiest when we feel in control, especially in regard to decisions affecting our own lives.

We authors are particularly interested in increasing the awareness of managers and counselors regarding stress and change for they significantly affect the lives of others. Much of the manager's energies are devoted to the management of *human* resources, and stress is a great waster of human resources. Its cost to business and industry now measures in the billions of dollars. It creates burnout, accidents, attention deficits, and performance failures. The courts now recognize the legitimacy of stress-induced disabilities. If managers are to manage human resources effectively, they often must manage stressed employees, and to do this best they must manage their own stress as well. Stressed-out managers often become stress spreaders, spreading stress like a contagion to their employees.

Counselors and therapists who have gained a keen understanding of stress will recognize its symptoms in the problems of their clients. We believe that stress is often a major contributor to marital disharmony, family discord, substance abuse, child and spousal abuse, mental illness, and many health problems. In the following pages we clearly trace the physiological basis for stress and stress-induced illness. We document the sources, symptoms, and treatments for stress. And by identifying the enabling conditions for change, we help counselors and therapists to discharge more fully their duties as change agents.

While we authors fully appreciate the significant contributions of counselors, therapists, and other professional helpers to the treatment of stress disorders, we do believe that persons often can successfully treat themselves for much of the warping from stress. Most people, however, are too ready to surrender responsibility for their stress and pain to professional fixers. They take their pained bodies to their doctors like they take their poorly running autos to the mechanic and say "I brought it, now you fix it!" They are like the young man who goes through the week sowing his wild oats and in church on Sunday prays for a crop failure. They are mostly interested in the "quick and dirty" ways of attending to the results of their stressful lifestyles. Instead of disciplining themselves into healthier lifestyles, they trust in psychopharmacological preparations to rid their symptoms. Valium is currently the fourth leading legal drug in this country. We are the most pill-popping, potion-guzzling group of people on earth. Contrary to public opinion, a headache is not the body's way of telling us we are short of aspirin. This child-like dependency on professional fixers and pharmaceutical preparations must be changed. In paraphrasing JFK we challenge the reader to "Ask not what your counselor, therapist, physician, or druggist can do for you, but what you can do for *yourself*!"

Most people have a deep-seated need to improve the quality of their lives — and this often entails changing their lifestyles to make them more stress free. Self-improvement requires the ability (a) to identify one's contribution to the stressful situations in one's life; (b) to uncover more functional ways of responding; (c) to focus attention on these more desirable behaviors in order to boost one's motivation for change; (d) to anticipate and accept beforehand the price we must pay for changing; and (e) to muster the energy necessary to follow through on difficult commitments. The suggestions offered in this volume will help the reader develop these abilities so necessary for redesigning one's lifestyle.

We offer at this point a word of caution to our readers. It is unwise to tie one's program for change to the efforts of others. If your plans for losing weight, taking up an exercise program, breaking the smoking habit, or learning to be more assertive, for example, depend on others to join you in the effort, your plan likely will fail. The journey into self-improvement is a lonely one. When the knights in King Arthur's court were setting out in search of the Holy Grail, one commented that it "would be a shame to go together." It is precisely because we must go it alone, because we must fall back on our own resources, on our own persistence, that success in self-improvement is so richly rewarding.

We further warn readers, however, not to expect miracles. It took many years to forge your present lifestyle, and change comes slowly — even with good maps and good strategies. Still, few feelings are more rewarding than the sense of personal power that comes from taking oneself in tow and successfully changing stress-inducing attitudes and behaviors.

We gratefully acknowledge the abundant assistance of many persons in readying this manuscript for publication. The staff of Georgia State University Business Press has been most helpful. In particular, Director R. Cary Bynum's enthusiasm and steady support has always been manifest. Margaret F. Stanley, Managing Editor, has greatly enhanced this work through her rigorous, always helpful, editorial review and general supervision. We also deeply appreciate the library research and steadfast commitment of Edith Jones. Finally, our students have reviewed and fine-tuned our efforts, and we are deeply appreciative of their contributions.

# PART I

# The Nature and Treatment of Stress

# CHAPTER ONE

# THE STRESS OF HELPLESSNESS

We lost because we told ourselves we lost.
——Leo Tolstoy, *War and Peace*

Healing does not rest in the hands of a selected few, but in the hands
of every human being . . . no matter what physicians do, they can only
augment the healing process of the body itself.
——W. B. Joy, *Joy's Way*

Stress and helplessness are like Siamese twins. Where you find one
you usually find the other. A life perceived to be out of control is a
stressful one. Research studies convincingly demonstrate the singular
importance of control in combating stress. It is mistakenly believed that
highly active persons are naturally highly stressed. However, the relationship between life events and stress actually is quite weak. Whether
events are experienced as stressful depends on the amount of control we
feel over them. Even a few events may prove stressful if we believe we
are inadequate to deal with them. In fact, heavy life demands may
actually strengthen one's defenses against stress and illness, *provided
one feels a sense of mastery over them.* As Nietzsche said, "What does
not destroy me, makes me stronger."

Stress is the result of a perception, the perception of helplessness in
facing serious demands. It is one's perception, and not the reality of the
situation, that determines whether life's demands will be experienced as
stressors or merely as challenges. Thus, there is no stress *out there!* Out
there are only people, places, and events; and whether we respond
stressfully to them depends on our perception of the adequacy of our
resources for dealing with them. We respond selectively to demands—

3

feeling powerful in dealing with some while helpless in dealing with others. Some of the demands we find most difficult are demands for self-regulation—demands to change our lifestyles in healthier directions.

Capable people, people who normally attack obstacles with exuberance, sometimes are wimps when confronting personal habits that direly need changing. They feel helpless when up against such habits as overeating, excessive drinking, smoking, procrastinating, or being hypercritical. This lack of *self*-control is not limited to the "little" people. Sharing this problem are members of the clergy, teachers, the captains of industry, politicians, and other movers and shakers among us. It is not the problem of the few, but of the many. When facing the burning need for self-control, our confidence sometimes melts, and left in its place is a depressing sense of resignation.

Why this astounding difference? Why the change from confidence to helplessness when facing personal problems? Perhaps our impotence stems from the belief that powerful forces hold us in their grip, and it is this fatalism that creates a pervasive sense of helplessness.

As long as we believe we cannot bring ourselves under control, we are likely to experience depression. Depression freezes us into a deadening state of apathy and lethargy. It will lift only when we change the belief that we are helpless to sculpture a healthier lifestyle. Our willingness to attack self-defeating habits is directly related to our perception of the probability of success. The following pages challenge the belief that we are helpless to change.

## Road Map for Change

Changing behavior is often a difficult process, and perhaps this is why at some level we are always ambivalent about attempting it. As indicated in Exhibit 1–1, the change process involves awareness, choice, and practice.

Change begins with awareness—awareness of the costs of harmful habits and awareness of alternative courses of action. We must consciously choose alternative behaviors and seriously commit ourselves to practice them. In time these replacement behaviors will become habits themselves. William James likened the forming of a new habit to the winding of string on a ball. The more string we wind without dropping it, the better. If we drop the string, we must spend time rewinding it.

**Exhibit 1-1.** Factors in the Process of Change

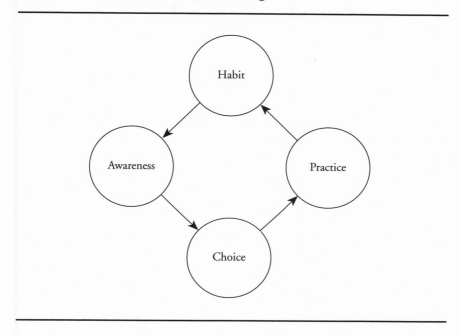

Like winding string, behaviors must be practiced again and again to make them habitual.

Self-theorists assert that we tend to behave in ways that are compatible with our self-concepts. How, then, do we form these internal guides to behavior? The social psychologist Daryl Bem contends that we get our self-concepts from what we see ourselves doing.[1] There is a circular relationship, therefore, between self-concepts and behavior. For example, persons who imagine themselves to be unable to change are *un*likely to engage in activities that would be needed to bring about the change. Other social psychologists emphasize the importance of significant others in determining our self-concepts. Charles Cooley held that our self-concepts come from our perception of how others see us.[2] Accordingly, we see ourselves as others see us. If early parental messages focused on our *in*abilities, we most likely will have learned to doubt our resources for coping. Once this self-doubt is in place, we thereafter are inclined to interpret our behaviors as failures, and in this way to develop more inadequate self-concepts. If we see ourselves as losers who are unable to change self-defeating behavioral patterns, we are unlikely to try seriously to change. Belief in powerful forces that control our behavior virtually eliminates any effort to change. We feel helpless, and this helplessness ultimately leads to depression.

## Interaction Between Stress and Depression

There exists a reciprocal relationship between stress and depression. Chronic stress often triggers depression, and depression from whatever source produces stress biochemicals. At any one time eight million Americans suffer from depression. Each year twenty-five thousand of them are driven to suicide. Depression is so epidemic that it has been called the common cold of psychiatry. George Washington and Abraham Lincoln both suffered from it. Fellow sufferer Winston Churchill referred to it as a "black dog." A line in Hamlet describes the feeling it causes: "How weary, stale, flat, and unprofitable seem to me all the uses of this world." Depression steals one's energy, diminishes one's interests, and flattens one's emotional life.

Depression erodes the quality of life, weakens the immune system, and decreases the life span. It alters the secretion of biochemicals affecting immunity. For example, cortisol, an adrenal hormone which is oversecreted by roughly half of all biologically depressed persons, is known to suppress immune functioning in five different ways!

### Types of Depression

Two forms of depression are widely acknowledged. One form, biological depression, is believed to result from flawed feedback systems which cause imbalances in brain chemicals. This form is most likely inherited and predisposes the person to multiple bouts of depression over a lifetime. While life circumstances may help trigger it at times, biological depression more often seems unrelated to life conditions. Medication often proves helpful with this form of depression.

Reactive depression, on the other hand, is a temporary response to stressful life situations. Bereavement is an excellent example of reactive depression. The typical widow may experience depression for up to three years and widowers, up to five years. Bereavement has been associated with the onset of diseases such as hypertension, rheumatoid arthritis, ulcers, and skin conditions.[3] Even more serious is the suppression of the immune system from the stress of bereavement. When rat pups are subjected to the loss of their mothers, their immune responses often function poorly *even in adulthood*. Because bereavement stress lasts so long, it is not surprising that the death rate for survivors in the year following the death of their spouses is many times greater than for other persons their same ages.

Current theory maintains that depression most likely results from an insufficiency of two classes of brain chemicals: neurotransmitters and endorphins. Neurotransmitters such as norepinephrine and serotonin allow brain cells to pass along messages. Norepinephrine activates reward centers in the brain; endorphins serve as pain killers and mood elevators. Severe depletion of norepinephrine and endorphins, therefore, would render a person incapable of fully experiencing rewarding sensations, and subsequently would produce anhedonia (lack of pleasure). Consequently, depressed persons would conclude that life holds little interest for them, that "vanity of vanities, all is vanity." This anhedonia is a universal symptom of depression.

Stress likely triggers depression by lowering the production of norepinephrine or endorphins. The triggering effect of stress upon depression is depicted in Exhibit 1–2. Stress from threats to one's well-being or frustration of strong needs increases the production of these biochemi-

**Exhibit 1–2.** Chronic Stress Triggers Depression

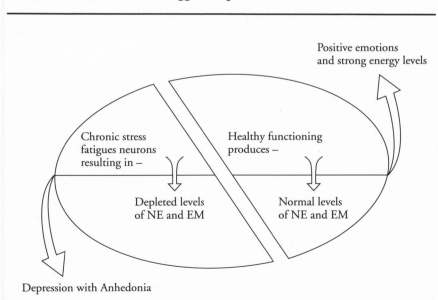

cals. If the stress is chronic, then severe depletion of these happiness chemicals may result from tissue fatigue. The physiologist Sherrington observed neuronal fatigue under chronic stress and referred to the phenomenon as reactive inhibition.[4] Neurons that are required to fire repeatedly for long periods produce metabolic deposits, which inhibit the further firing of these neurons. After the deposits dissipate, the neurons recover their ability to fire. When tissues producing norepinephrine and endorphins are fatigued, reward centers are understimulated and the person is thrust into depression while the brain tissue is recovering.

If the condition is not worsened by negative thinking, the depression will lift of itself within days as the production of these biochemicals return to normal levels. Negative thinking, however, can sustain and aggravate the depressive reaction. Thoughts are made up of reverberating circuits of brain cells, called neurons. A single thought may involve tens of thousands of these neurons. Some of the branches of these neurons, called axons, extend downward from the cortex to limbic structures within the emotional part of the brain. Neurons stimulating a limbic structure called the amygdala cause it to incite the stress response. Neurons stimulating another limbic structure called the septo-hippocampal system, on the other hand, trigger positive emotions. If one's thinking is made up of neurons extending to the amygdala, one's mood will be heavy and somber. However, thinking comprised of neurons terminating in the septo-hippocampal system induces pleasant emotions. Negative thinking, then, produces stressful emotional reactions, which may further deplete norepinephrine and endorphins, and in this way sustains the depressive reaction. Exhibit 1–3 depicts the role of negative thinking in aggravating depression.

It is important for depressed persons to understand that their depression is a natural outcome of the depletion of these upbeat biochemicals, that the condition is temporary, and that they will recover automatically as the production of these biochemicals return to normal levels. They should realize that at this point there is nothing to be done but merely to cope until the biochemistry changes. Understanding this process will allay fears that the condition is permanent. While awaiting the restoration of the tissue's ability to resume production of norepinephrine and endorphins, the following coping strategy may be helpful:

- Do not try to hide your depression from your spouse, children, or closest friends. Otherwise, they may misinterpret your feelings to be anger directed toward them. Letting them know that

**Exhibit 1-3.** Negative Thoughts Generate Stress Which Intensifies Depression

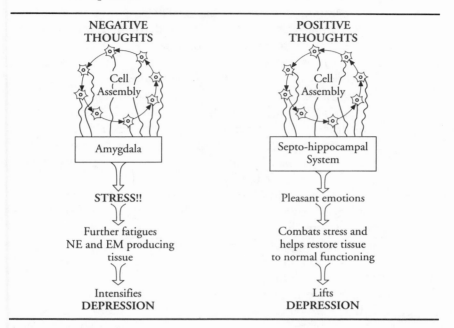

you are slipping into a depressive episode may keep them from becoming defensive with you and head off strained interpersonal relationships. Interpersonal problems on top of the depression only creates more depression.

- Lower your self-expectations temporarily. Do jobs that do not require much mental energy. If you are a perfectionist, require only 80 percent of yourself instead of the usual 100 percent. Realize that you are not being lazy—you are only working with the *temporarily* impaired condition of the human machine.
- While you will not feel like doing so, exercise may do wonders for you at this time. Moderate exercise releases endorphins which elevate the mood. Experiment with exercise as a treatment. You may be pleasantly surprised with the temporary relief which the endorphins produce. A rewarding side effect is the sense of control over the depression which accompanies the use of this healthy practice.
- Reward yourself for coping with your depression. Plan ahead as

to what you can do to reward yourself on those days that you feel depressed. Think of activities you can do that do not require extensive interaction with others, such as going to a movie, concert, or ball game. When depressed, then, reward yourself with one of these activities. The rationale behind this practice is that your depression will be relieved more quickly if you accept it and cope with it than if you try to ignore it.

- Continuously remind yourself that your condition is transient. Tell yourself "This too shall pass!" It is temporarily beyond your control. It is not a problem to be solved; rather, it is a condition with which you must cope. There is nothing to be done. You should treat yourself kindly, deal with your symptoms as best you can, and wait for the depression to lift.

- Feed your depression properly. Tendencies toward excessive eating or loss of appetite may peak during depression because the body is incorrectly trying to find different solutions to its biochemical imbalance and the mind's problems. Fight this by forcing yourself to monitor with special vigilance the intake of fluid and fiber for its nutritional adequacy.

- If suffering from biological depression, you need to accept the fact that your feeling state is the result of biological changes presently beyond your control. Acknowledge that you need medication for your condition in the same way that the diabetic needs insulin. However, remind yourself that you can live with the condition satisfactorily if you cope wisely.

While this approach may be less than perfect, it is a way of approaching depression that is positive and somewhat hopeful. It does offer a kind of structure, and structure is often useful when dealing with feelings of helplessness.

## Diagnosing Depression

Diagnosing the difference between biological and reactive depression is not an easy matter. Indeed, most depressions are a mixture of the two because each form predisposes the other. In making the diagnosis biopsychiatrists usually test for serum levels of cortisol and/or thyroid stimulating hormone. Levels of these hormones are kept within a narrow range by cooperative action from the hypothalamus, the pituitary, and adrenal or thyroid glands. Exhibit 1–4 graphically displays the relationships among these endocrine glands and their hormones. Even the

**Exhibit 1-4.** Feedback Systems Regulating Production of Cortisol and Thyroxin

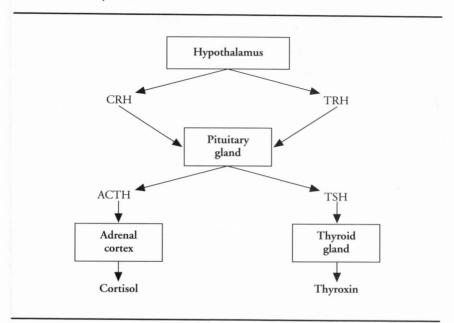

smallest alterations in their secretion can significantly upset the balance required for normal brain functioning. In most cases of biological depression these hormone levels are abnormal. Depressives often overproduce these hormones even when the glands that produce them are themselves normal. This suggests a problem with the regulation mechanism for these hormones.

The hypothalamus plays a critical role in regulating the production of both cortisol and thyroxin. It regulates levels of *cortisol* through the production of corticotropic-releasing hormone (CRH). This hormone regulates the production of adrenocorticotropic hormone (ACTH) by the pituitary gland, which in turn regulates the production of cortisol by the adrenal glands. The hypothalamus monitors the serum level of cortisol. If too much or too little is detected, it adjusts the production of CRH. This regulatory system can be challenged by injecting dexamethasone, a synthetic version of cortisol, into the patient's blood stream to see if the hypothalamus will adjust for the excess concentration of cortisol by lowering its production of CRH. This test is referred to as the

DST, the dexamethasone suppression test. About 50 percent of depressives fail this test; that is the hypothalamus does not lower the production of CRH to lessen the production of cortisol. The test is not conclusive, however, as the results sometimes prove positive even when there is no depression. In such cases it is presumed that another illness has caused the regulatory failure.

The hypothalamus also regulates levels of *thyroxin* by producing more or less of a thyroid-releasing hormone (TRH). TRH is picked up in the pituitary gland, causing it to produce more thyroid stimulating hormone (TSH), which in turn, stimulates the thyroid gland to produce more thyroxin. To check for depression, TRH is injected to see if the pituitary will adjust its production of TSH. This test is referred to as the TRH stimulation test. Mark Gold claims that the DST and TRH tests together can identify biological malfunction in approximately 85 percent of unipolar depressives.[5]

Michael Gazzaniga suggests two other bases for distinguishing between biological and situational depression.[6] He notes that antidepressive medications do little to lift situational depression. Furthermore, he points out that situational depressives will respond with enthusiasm when asked if they would like to move out of their current situation, whereas biologically based depressives will indicate that it does not matter.

## Other Causes of Depression

*Repressed Anger.* Psychoanalytic theory maintains that depression often results from repressed anger which gets redirected toward oneself. Depressed persons are said to be afraid to direct their anger toward the actual source, and so they turn it inward on themselves. According to this theory, the proper treatment of depression requires the working through of repressed anger.

*Patterns of Thinking.* Cognitive therapists believe depression is a natural consequence of pessimistic beliefs and illogical patterns of thinking. Aaron Beck identifies three dysfunctional themes in the thinking of depressives.[7] These themes, referred to as the *cognitive triad,* include the belief that one is no good, that others are not worth much either, and that one's situation is not likely to get better. Depressives are said to magnify the seriousness of demands, to generalize the negative results from small events to broader vistas in their lives, and to make arbitrary, unpleasant inferences about themselves from events going on around them.

*Misfiring of Brain Cells.* Gazzaniga claims that depression, as well as other forms of mental illness, is triggered by capricious misfiring of brain cells and is often reinforced by an overlay of neurotic thinking which develops to explain these random changes in behavior and effect.[8] Because persons have no understanding of the biological causes of their depression, they create explanations for it. These explanations are sometimes elaborate and usually neurotic. Once in place these beliefs further aggravate the depression. While antidepressive medications often smooth out the neuronal misfiring, the negative thinking patterns may remain to single-handedly maintain the depression. It is a well-known fact that persons suffering from depression are best helped early in their disease—probably because early intervention interrupts the consolidation of such neurotic beliefs. Biochemical remedies that typically work well are not always effective for the hardened depressed patient.

*Diminishing Light Intensities.* Recently the role of diminishing natural light in triggering depression has been uncovered. The brain's pineal gland monitors light intensity. When the light source dims and darkness increases, this gland increases the production of melatonin, a hibernation-like drug that slows neurotransmission. It is quite likely that natural selection bred-in this reaction to assist our ancestors in enduring the long, dark winters with their scarce food supplies. Inducing sluggishness in metabolic functioning would lower food requirements and increase one's chances of surviving. Depression has been associated in some persons with increased levels of melatonin. Such persons are said to suffer from SAD, seasonally affective disorder. Symptoms, other than hibernation lethargy, experienced by SAD patients include large appetite and overeating, weight gain, and carbohydrate craving. Treatment for SAD is very simple. Merely expose the depressive to more light. Spend winters in the Caribbean or sit in front of a bank of lights five to ten times more intense than usual indoor light for three hours at the beginning and end of the day.

*Helplessness.* From years of studying the "helplessness syndrome," Martin Seligman concluded that helplessness leads to panic and panic to depression.[9] Looking more carefully at the helplessness syndrome, Abramson, Seligman, and Teasdale concluded that the syndrome is learned only when persons are exposed to unpredictable negative events *and yet* attribute their emotional reactions to personal traits.[10] This describes the experience of the children who fault themselves for the punishment given them capriciously by dysfunctional parents. Feeling little control over their punishment, these children are likely to learn that their behavior does not matter since the punishment seems unrelated to it. This helpless attitude is crippling when the person experiences personal needs. When strong needs are chronically frustrated, drive states rise to panicky proportions. If the person loses hope of ever meeting these needs, the panic trails off into depression. Exhibit 1–5 depicts the relationship among these variables.

The exhibit suggests that our activity level is energetic and our feeling tone is confident when we feel resourceful. Even moderate degrees of helplessness, however, lead to an agitated activity level and an anxious feeling state. Further helplessness turns agitation into mania and anxiety into panic. The psychic pain accompanying these states may thrust us into depression and lethargy as a means of lessening the serious wear and tear inflicted by sustained mania and panic. Viewed in this way, depression is a self-protective process that shuts down potentially overworked systems in the interest of damage control. It would be much healthier yet if depressives employed the energy used in this manner to direct their own lives.

**Exhibit 1–5.** The Effects of Helplessness

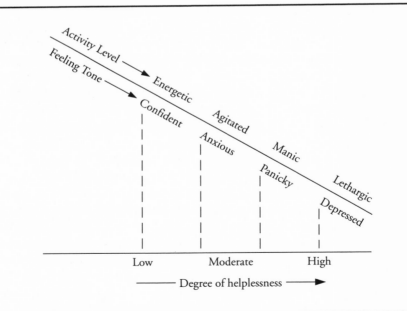

## Control — An Effective Buffer Against Stress and Depression

While helplessness generates stress, a sense of control prevents it. Some studies suggest that the mere *perception* of control is enough to prevent the stress response. Medicine has made ample use of placebos — inactive substances used to cause patients to believe they were getting help. In reviewing placebo studies Blair Justice concludes that any intervention that enhances positive expectations and a sense of control can trigger the placebo response, and, contrary to what is commonly assumed about the use of placebos, *no deceit is necessary.*[11] In one study all but one patient showed improvement in a week when told that sugar pills they were to be given had helped others and might help them. In another study hypertensive patients, told that the regular monitoring of their blood pressure would reduce the pressure, experienced the placebo effect upon adopting the practice of taking their own blood pressure. The placebo response appears to depend on faith in one's ability to control the bad condition rather than on whatever pill one might take. Justice states: "Whatever gives us an increased sense of control — whether it's love, faith, or cognitive coping — seems to mobilize our self-healing process . . . The real scene, real war, the new frontier is the internal environment."

## Biochemical Treatments for Depression

The treatments for depression generally are more successful than for other forms of mental distress. If treated early, most types of biological depression respond well to medication. Medication comes in three classes: tricyclicates, MAO inhibitors, and lithium. The first two classes are aimed at *increasing* the effects of biochemicals that activate the brain's reward centers, while lithium is used to balance the action of electrolytes.

In order for brain cells, called neurons, to pass along their messages, small amounts of neurotransmitters, like norepinephrine and serotonin, are released at the terminals of the neuron's axons into a microscopically small area (about one millionth of an inch) between two neurons, called a synapse. These chemicals are picked up by receptor cells on the surface of nearby neurons. If enough of these chemicals are picked up, the receiving nerve cell sends its message along to yet other neurons. The higher the concentration of the neurotransmitter and the longer it stays in the synapse the greater the likelihood that the adjacent neuron will fire and continue the message chain.

*Tricyclicates.* As a conservation measure, part of the neurotransmitter substance is pumped back into the sending neuron, a process called "re-uptake," to prepare it to send future messages. Tricyclicates, such as amitriptyline (Elavil), retard the re-uptake of norepinephrine and serotonin. This allows for a greater concentration of these neurotransmitters for a longer time in the synapse, thus increasing the probability that the receiving neuron will continue the message chain. Because norepinephrine and serotonin activate reward pathways in the brain, increasing their effects in this manner typically lifts the mood state of the depressive.

*MAO Inhibitors.* Norepinephrine and serotonin in the synapse are broken down slowly by monoamine oxidase (MAO). MAO inhibitors, such as Nardil, slow the breakdown and, thus, increase the amount of these neurotransmitters within the synapses. In this manner the action of these rewarding neurotransmitters is enhanced once again.

*Lithium.* Electrolytes such as sodium, calcium, potassium, and magnesium assist in the transmission of messages across synapses. Imbalances in these electrolytes appear in certain types of depression. Lithium, a simple salt, often works wonders in balancing the action of these electrolytes. In this way it boosts the effectiveness of the reward transmitters norepinephrine and serotonin. It seems to increase their effectiveness when they are in short supply and to decrease their effectiveness when they are overly abundant. Lithium is particularly effective in treating mania, the agitated half of the bipolar depressive syndrome.

This brief discussion of psychopharmaceutical agents is grossly incomplete as there are other biochemical agents currently being researched that have not been mentioned. The biological treatments are multiple and varied, and many factors must be considered in their prescription; however, these agents have proven helpful to thousands of depressives.

## Psychological Treatment

Currently the predominant psychological treatment of depression is cognitive in orientation. Cognitive therapists believe that thinking patterns initiate or worsen the depressive code and must be changed. Gazzaniga asserts that psychopharmacology *and* psychological treatments must be combined in treating biological depression.[12] The psychopharmaceutical agents may return balance to biochemical functioning, but the belief system created to explain the patient's symptoms remains and must be challenged for lasting results. In addition to efforts to rid the client of irrational, self-defeating thoughts, cognitive therapists encourage depressed clients to behave more forcefully. They are urged to make choices, assert themselves, and, in general, remind themselves of the many areas of their lives where they are in charge. It is not so much a matter of gaining control as it is of *acknowledging* the control they already have. This requires directing their attention to personal successes and strengths. The goal is personal empowerment, to increase their sense of resourcefulness to counter their sense of helplessness.

At the very least, helplessness is an accompaniment of depression. It springs from the conviction that forces over which we have no control determine our behavior. These forces may be seen as some kind of internal intrapsychical power that derives from the cumulative effects of past conditioning or from current physical and social pressures.

## The Enemy Within

Since we are sometimes mystified by the nature of our problems, we are often tempted to believe that they originate from an unrecognized internal source. There are, in fact, views within religion and psychiatry to foster this belief. The Calvinist concept of original sin and the modern Freudian concept of the unconscious both suggest that the biggest barrier to personal development is within. In reference to the influence of original sin upon his behavior, St. Paul concluded, "I do not understand my own actions, for I do not do what I want, but I do the very thing I hate" (Romans 7:15, Revised Standard Version). Freud suggested that behavior is more determined by unconscious drives than by conscious ones. He used the metaphor of an iceberg to make his point. The conscious was likened to the small tip of an iceberg, with the unconscious as its huge submerged base. Accordingly, the actual causes of our actions are said to be deeply submerged in the unconscious. In both Calvinist theology and Freudian psychology we are portrayed as puppets whose strings are pulled by some puppeteer. It helps little that the puppeteer is some unfathomable power within us, since it is a power that eludes our will.

Behavior is undoubtedly influenced to some degree by desires and impulses that we do not understand. Few people would suggest that they are perfectly aware of *all* of the reasons for their behavior. The role of the unconscious appears to be considerably more influential in the behavior of seriously disturbed people. Anxiety-arousing impulses and painful memories may be relegated to the unconscious when we have given up hope of successfully coping with them, but this model of unconscious determination of behavior fits less well the functioning of the normal person. Normal persons are more aware of what they are doing. They are creatures of habit, however, and habits are not broken easily; nevertheless, they will give way to well-designed, persistent efforts to change them.

# The Tyranny of the Past

In Homer's *Odyssey,* Odysseus says, "I am part of all that I have met." This was Homer's way of emphasizing the important influence of past experience in shaping us. Odysseus bore the imprint of former battles, of far-flung travels, and intoxicating romantic episodes. Like Odysseus, all people carry the imprint of past experiences. Relationships within the family, formal schooling, work experiences, and chance acquaintances all have their influences.

Even emotional responses often are shaped through past experiences. Frequently associating emotionally neutral experiences with ones that evoke strong emotion will gradually invest them with the ability to evoke the same strong response. Such associations form the basis for prejudiced thinking. The targets of racial prejudice are presented in negative contexts so often that they come to trigger negative feelings. Consequently, feelings are not necessarily the best guide to behavior, since they merely reflect earlier emotional conditioning that may or may not be functional. Once we become aware of such emotional conditioning, we can recondition ourselves by making new and favorable associations with the target of the prejudice.

Past experience also provides a set of beliefs, expectations, and assumptions through which future experiences are viewed. We see the world from our unique perspectives, and what we see at times may be but a pale reflection of reality. We are judging creatures. We seldom have an experience without evaluating it, and the basis for this evaluation comes from the quality of past experience. These beliefs and expectations serve as sunglasses that color our experiences—good or bad, promising or ominous.

Once we become aware of these restricting beliefs and expectations, we can open ourselves to new experiences and, thus, revise our views to make them conform more closely to reality. We will be slaves to archaic thoughts *only* if we fail to surface them so they can be challenged.

While the past influences present behavior, it is possible to overemphasize its importance to such an extent that we become convinced that personal change is impossible. For example, we can come to believe that bad homes, bad parents, or bad love experiences have condemned us to live our days in helpless enslavement to these influences. Yet such a view does not conform with the facts because, as Exhibit 1–1 shows, awareness can lead to choice, choice can lead to the practice of new behaviors, and repeated practice can lead to the creation of more functional habits.

## Environmental Influences

Our sense of personal helplessness is often aggravated by *overestimating* the controlling influence of pressures in the environment. There is no denying that people are influenced by the responses of others, but it seems an overstatement to say that they are *controlled* by them.

Some behavioral scientists are fond of saying that behavior is governed by its consequences; that is to say, that people tend to repeat behaviors that are rewarding and to drop those that are punishing. In an NBC Special Report entitled *The Blue Collar Trap,* an automotive worker complained that he was being paid too well. He felt the pay for his labor was such that he could not afford to quit despite his total distaste for the work. He saw himself as a gigolo whose body was bought with a handsome wage. He felt he was hooked on the rewarding consequences of his distasteful work.

There are two ways of looking at these consequences. They may be seen as shaping behavior, or the behavior may be seen as being their cause. Both views are accurate. We are modified by our environment, but we also modify it. The factory worker was encouraged to continue his distasteful work in order to earn his wage, but he caused his wage to be paid precisely because he did his work. In this ultimate sense, he chose to continue his work. People often choose their own conditioners. They may complain that others influence them to eat too much, but they have *chosen* their company. A student may protest that he would study more if his crowd were not so socially minded, and yet he *chooses* to run with them. A woman may complain that it is almost impossible to keep from losing her temper when she plays bridge with her neighbor, and yet she *chooses* to play with this person.

We can choose more positive influences on our behavior and mood states. This may involve selecting different friends, a different occupation, a different school, or even a different spouse. Sometimes, we may choose to maintain these associations because they contribute significantly to our happiness in some other way. In this case we are still free to choose our attitudes toward these conditioners. We are free to attach great or little significance to the barbs of others. Conversely, we can often see through the manipulative praise of others and refuse to be swayed from a position based on our best judgment.

The nobel laureate Roger Sperry, from the California Institute of Technology, wrote that science has a blind spot: it has ignored the area of subjective human experience.[13] In his view, science fails to appreciate the power of human thoughts in influencing the course of history. He maintains that serious thinkers are leaving behind the determinism, behaviorism, and the materialism of the past. These brands of science have been useful, but today we recognize *the primacy of inner conscious awareness as a causal reality.* That phrase is dynamite! Very simply it means that our minds affect reality, that the inner decisions we make influence our actions and thereby have an effect on our environment. In this sense we are creating our own reality. It is empowering to shift from thinking we are victims to the idea that we can materially affect what is going on with our minds. There is evidence that we can use the mind to regulate athletic performance, the heart rate, our blood pressure, and sometimes it can effect miraculous turn-arounds in terminal illness. It appears that we have grossly underestimated our own powers—our ability to materially affect our environment.

We may feel helpless if we fail to see that our behavior is causing the consequence. If what happens appears to be the result of luck, fate, or chance, rather than the natural result of our behavior, then feelings of helplessness and confusion may result, and we may see ourselves as pawns in the hands of some unfathomable, unpredictable force.

Most of the time, though, a logical connection exists between what happens and the behavior that precedes an event. It is true that some people have been subjected to bad parenting in which rewards and punishments were handed out in a whimsical, capricious manner. They were punished for actions for which they were rewarded at other times. Children coming out of such environments feel that nothing they do will make any difference. The effect of this kind of conditioning is best seen in an experiment by Seligman and his associates. They subjected a group of dogs to inconsistently presented shock. At first these dogs responded normally by defecating, urinating, barking, and straining against their harnesses. They soon discovered that nothing they did influenced the shocks, and thereafter, they stopped these futile efforts and passively accepted their fate. In a second experimental setting, where half the floor was wired for electrical discharges and the other half was not, these same dogs failed to escape their punishment even though their harnesses had been removed. The external harnesses had been replaced with an equally binding internal harness. They had learned a sense of helplessness by coming to believe that there was no relationship between what they did and what happened to them.[14]

In much the same way, many people have developed a helplessness syndrome that strongly influences their behavior. It is important to understand that helplessness comes not from our experiences but from what we come to believe about them. We carry these beliefs, and they are just as binding as the dogs' harnesses. Therapists generally agree that among the most shackling of beliefs are the following:

- *It is dangerous to have others unhappy with me.* Children who have suffered parental abuse may have maintained this belief long after it ceased to be functional. As adults they may become frightened when others become angry with them. They may go to great lengths to keep others from getting angry, and they may placate them when they do. Consequently, such people are seldom true to themselves, since they fashion their views according to the reception they get from others. They haven't yet learned that it is impossible to maintain a sense of integrity and still have everyone happy with them at *all* times.

- *I should feel guilty about past mistakes.* People spend considerable time rehearsing their past mistakes. While it is obvious that they can do nothing about them, they nevertheless persist in blaming themselves. Perhaps they believe that self-criticism will deter others from attacking them. Unfortunately, this focusing on past mistakes robs them of the energy for present pursuits and renders them overly cautious.

- *I should constantly anticipate all the potential dangers of the future.* People who believe this are afraid of the future and try to shove it into the past by constantly rehearsing for it. Each time we needlessly worry about the future, we give ourselves a vote of "No Confidence." Because we distrust our coping resources, we experience stage fright when facing the future. The resulting cautiousness destroys the rhythm of spontaneous living. One colleague calls needless worrying "building bridges over rivers God hasn't even made yet."

- *I should be competent in all aspects of my life.* Many of us exaggerate the importance of making mistakes, of being less than perfect. We lack the courage to be *im*perfect. Perfectionism is brittle. It leaves us humorless and overly intense. It inhibits us from experimenting with new behaviors and new tastes and limits us to those tasks wherein we are assured of success.

• *I must be happy all the time and if I'm not it's someone else's fault.* One of the most frequent errors in personal logic is to charge others with the responsibility for one's happiness. Husbands blame wives, wives blame husbands, children blame parents, parents blame children. This error in logic is the cause of enormous suffering in relationships. Projecting the responsibility for our misery on others is self-deluding. Real progress begins only when we accept responsibility for our happiness.

These neurotic beliefs create a defensiveness, a cautiousness, a fearfulness about behavior that is just as binding as any external harness. In holding these beliefs, we become mere shadows of the people we could be if our risk-taking were greater.

Seldom are human beings subjected to conditions as extreme as those to which the dogs in the Seligman and Maier study were subjected. Occasionally, however, human beings find themselves subjected to inhumane conditions, but even then they are free to determine their reactions to such conditions. Victor Frankl was interred in a Nazi concentration camp and lived to write about it:

> We who lived in concentration camps can remember the men who walked through the huts comforting others, giving away their last piece of bread. They may have been few in number, but they offer sufficient proof that everything can be taken from a man but one thing: the last of the human freedoms — to choose one's attitude in any given set of circumstances, to choose one's own way.[15]

Once we perceive the connection between behavior and its consequences, we realize that we can change the consequences by changing our behavior. To some extent, then, we are responsible for what happens to us because we are free to change the behavior that brings about a given consequence.

Quite often the most important consequences influencing behavior are thoughts and are not part of the external environment. People often reward or punish themselves for actions that either aid or hinder them in pursuing personal goals, and these self-endorsing or self-criticizing thoughts are often more influential than those stemming from outside sources. These powerful self-rewards and self-punishments can be changed with effort.

In summary, while the physical and social environments influence our behavior, these influences are often countered or abetted by self-endorsing or self-critical thoughts. We are influenced by the external environment, but we influence it in turn, and are capable of modifying its influence further by the attitudes that we adopt toward it.

## Running from Responsibility

The Danish philosopher Kierkegaard once said, "Anxiety is the price of freedom." Feeling free, and therefore responsible, makes us nervous. Growing and changing often involve giving up familiar sources of nourishment to search for more rewarding sources in much the same way that an infant must give up the nourishing placenta to experience the freedom of the outside world. When we feel the need for change, yet allow feelings of helplessness to immobilize us, the result is personal stagnation, self-contempt, and depression.

Personal change is often forged on a crucible of suffering. When we say, "I can't change," often we mean, "I won't change." Growth is frequently painful, and people conveniently adopt beliefs that excuse them from trying. As a result of these beliefs, our growth is severely stunted. William James wrote, "Compared with what we ought to be, we are only half awake. Our fires are dampened, our drafts are checked. We are making use of only a small part of our mental and physical resources."[16]

If we are to take responsibility for what we are and for what happens to us, we must give up favorite villains such as the unconscious, traumatic past experiences, poor parents, the expectations of significant others, and family responsibilities. What these forces can do is insignificant when compared with the effects of crippling personal beliefs. In George Bernard Shaw's *Mrs. Warren's Profession,* one of the characters says:

> People are always blaming their circumstance for what they are. I don't believe in circumstances. The people who get on in this world are the people who get up and look for the circumstances they want, and if they can't find them, make them.[17]

This book contains many starting places for people wishing to take charge of their lives. The authors invite readers to select as targets for change the behaviors they have long wished to learn, unlearn, or modify.

This book is written in the belief that striving can be as satisfying as achieving, that people are most happy when they feel they are improving in some way that seems important. We do not have to change in an all-or-nothing fashion. Gradual improvement in some small sphere can be exhilarating and furnish the motivation for further improvement. Perhaps the most significant result of self-engineered change is the thrilling sense of control over ourselves. For many, the new frontier is internal, and conquests there are the most rewarding of all.

The reader should not expect magical cures in the following pages. The authors have yet to stumble on any such tonic. Growth is a dividend yielded by the investment of energy and self. Perhaps no other key is as crucial as is the old-fashioned idea of involvement. And perhaps there is no sounder contribution to our mental health than the kind of authorship over our own life that dispels a sense of personal helplessness.

> And will you succeed?
> Yes! You will, indeed!
> (98 and 3/4 percent guaranteed.)"
> ——Dr. Seuss (1990)

## ENDNOTES

1. Daryl J. Bem, "Self-perception Theory," *Advances in Experimental Social Psychology, vol. 6*, ed. L. Berkowitz (New York: Academic Press, 1972).

2. Charles Cooley, *Social Organization* (New York: Scribner's, 1937).

3. Mark S. Gold and Lois B. Morris, *The Good News About Depression* (New York: Bantam, 1986).

4. C. S. Sherrington, *Integrative Action of the Nervous System* (New Haven, Connecticut: Yale University Press, 1906).

5. Gold and Morris, *Good News.*

6. Michael S. Gazzaniga, *Mind Matters: How Mind and Brain Interact to Create Our Consciousness* (Boston: Houghton Mifflin, 1988).

7. Aaron T. Beck, *Cognitive Therapy and the Emotional Disorders* (New York: International Universities Press, 1976).

8. Gazzaniga, *Mind Matters.*

9. Martin E. Seligman, *Helplessness: On Depression, Development, and Death* (San Francisco: W. H. Freeman, 1975).

10. L. Y. Abramson, M. E. P. Seligman, and J. D. Teasdale, "Learned Helplessness in Humans: Critique and Formulation," *Journal of Abnormal Psychology* 87, no. 1 (1978).

11. Blair Justice, *Who Gets Sick* (Los Angeles: Jeremy P. Tarcher, 1988).

12. Gazzaniga, *Mind Matters*.

13. Roger Sperry, "Psychology's Mentalist Paradigm and Religion/Science Tension," *American Psychologist* 43, no. 8 (1988), 607–613.

14. Seligman, *Helplessness*.

15. Victor Frankl, *Man's Search for Meaning* (New York: Beacon, 1959), 12.

16. William James, *Varieties of Religious Experience* (New York: Random House, Modern Library, 1902).

17. George Bernard Shaw, *Mrs. Warren's Profession* (Hamden, Connecticut: Garland, 1981).

# CHAPTER TWO

# UNDERSTANDING THE STRESS IN DISTRESS

Imitate the sundial's ways;
Count only the pleasant days.
——German proverb

Stress is public enemy number 1! It exacts a frightful price. It contributes to the absenteeism, job dissatisfaction, interpersonal conflict, escalating insurance premiums, and failing performance. Stress-related accidents cost American business and industry approximately $100 billion annually. Moreover, stress constitutes a serious threat to our health. It is a contributing factor to heart disease, strokes, ulcers, hypertension, rheumatoid arthritis, mental illness and a host of other diseases.

In 1991 Americans spent over $800 billion on the nation's health bill. Approximately 70 percent of the illnesses that contribute to this bill are degenerative, not infectious, diseases. Degenerative diseases are referred to as lifestyle diseases due to the critical role that habits and mental attitudes play in bringing them on. We are not so much sick of microbes as we are of unhealthy lifestyles, and contributing significantly to such lifestyles is mismanaged stress.

Stress is the body's reflexive response to stressors, that is, to anything perceived to be frustrating or dangerous. The danger may be real or imagined; it doesn't matter. The perception triggers the stress response with its powerful stress hormones and lightning-like shifts in the nervous system. It was bred into us eons ago when life for humans on this planet was full of jeopardy. Our ancestors were stalked by tigers in the jungles and lions on the savannahs, and they had no technology to protect them from the elements. For the longest time survival for them was a matter of serious question. Hypervigilant humans survived, while the laid-back types were eaten up; thus, the only members left to pass along the gene pool were the nervous Nellies—those humans with nervous systems honed to hair-trigger sensitivity.

Physical dangers have decreased markedly throughout our history, but there is little evidence that our nervous systems are evolving into less hyper, healthier ones.[1] This hypervigilant nervous system that was the salvation of our ancestors eons ago, is now an evolutionary hangover. In one sense this vestigial legacy from the distant past is our greatest *enemy*! The ultimate in stress management, therefore, may be the taming of our hypervigilant and pugnacious nervous systems.

In most cases the stress response is a greater threat to one's health than the perceived threat that triggers it. The stress response is somewhat analogous to an allergic reaction. The allergen triggering the allergic reaction presents no real threat to the person's well-being. The body's unnecessary defense reaction, the allergic response, however, *is* a threat. It results in swollen membranes, mucous discharge, and inflammation. Similarly, most stress responses are totally unnecessary. Most situations that trigger the stress response are perceived threats to our *egos,* not to our bodies, and the fight-flight readiness of the stress response is counterproductive in handling such threats. At the least, the unnecessary arousal accompanying the stress response interferes with clear thinking, is a waste of our energy, and a drain on our emotions. At worst, it imperils our health, lowers our work performance, interrupts our relationships with others, and, in general, erodes the quality of our lives.

## Mismanaging Stressors Becomes Costly

These days we encounter very few tigers in the jungles. The modern equivalent of the tiger is the supervisor who berates us in the presence of fellow employees. In our mind's eye the supervisor turns into a raging tiger; consequently our bodies pump out stress hormones and initiate massive changes in our neurology to prepare us to club the beast to death or turn and run like sprinters. Typically the stress does not go away when the supervisor goes away. Rather, we return to our work stations and unsuccessfully try to distract our attention from the embarrassment. Unfortunately, our minds return to the scene of the crime repeatedly, and each time our bodies experience the stress response. We rehearse and re-rehearse this hurtful scene. We may repeat it twenty times before leaving for home, and each time we trigger the stress response because *the body doesn't know the difference between fact and fantasy!* Whatever the mind pictures, the body treats as reality.

Most persons *mis*manage these threats to their egos. As just suggested, they endlessly rehearse the humiliation and soon are partially inebriated on their stress hormones. Because these hormones were meant to be dissipated by vigorous action such as running or fighting, and because our work is typically sedentary, the stress hormones cascade to dangerous heights, and we are filled with strong emotion. We pack it in and pack it in like gun powder down the muzzle of an old musket.

Typically we hold onto our anger in such situations in order to save our jobs. Later, however, we may dump it on family members or friends. Metaphorically speaking, we walk onto the porch with smoke curling out of our ears. The furry cat wraps itself around our foot, and we send it off chasing comets. We don't bother to open the door, we walk through it. We spread stress to the right, to the left, in front of us, and behind us. Before the evening is over everyone in the household is infected with the stress contagion. Through our failure to manage the stress, we become stress spreaders for others.

Stress destroys a sense of personal well-being. It often ruptures interpersonal relationships and contributes to the painfully high divorce rate that presently approaches 40 percent. It is a significant factor in causing roughly one out of every ten Americans to experience a serious mental or emotional breakdown and millions to suffer from alcohol and other drug addictions. It contributes to headaches and backaches, which erode the quality of living. Pain signals from such conditions are nature's way of telling us something is wrong with our lifestyles.

Unfortunately, we Americans tend to ignore pain signals rather than take the corrective action they call for; or worse yet, we mask such signals with pharmacological aids. For, after all, in the words of a current commercial jingle, "We haven't got time for the pain." Contrary to common opinion, however, a headache is *not* the body's way of telling us it's running out of aspirin! Rather than do the hard work of changing our lifestyles, we depend on analgesics and tranquilizers to mute the pain.

A certain amount of stress is unavoidable, and some stress is even healthy. Hans Selye referred to such stress as *eustress*.[2] An automobile engine experiences less wear when running at moderate speeds than when idling. Similarly, the human body may experience less wear when under moderate pressure than when subjected to *enforced inactivity*. Most people, however, live with far more stress than is healthy. Mishandling stress only adds to the problem. Stress is mishandled when we allow demands made on us to exact a greater price in adaptive energy than is necessary. Consequently, it is important that we learn to cope *efficiently* with stressors.

# Perception Is the Key

Stress is not an *external* reality. There is no stress *out there*. It is all inside our heads. It is not what happens to us that causes us stress but rather our perception of what is happening. An anonymous writer sums up the relationship between perception and reality:

> Projection makes perception. The world you see is what you gave it, nothing more than that. . . .It is the witness to your state of mind, the outside picture of an inward condition. As a man thinketh, so does he perceive. Therefore, seek not to change the world, but choose to change your mind about the world.

## The Role of Appraisal

Modern theories view stress as the inequality between *perceived* demands and *perceived* resources. The stress model presented in Exhibit 2–1 depicts the critical role of appraisal in turning demands into stressors. The process begins with demands either from self-requirements, life changes, roles we play, or hassles. Awareness of these demands is followed by appraisal of their severity and importance (primary appraisal) and the adequacy of resources for coping with them (secondary appraisal).[3] If resources seem adequate for coping with the demands, the demands are viewed as challenges and we deal with them healthily. If, however, demands seem too great for our resources, they become stressors and trigger the stress response with its three classes of symptoms.

The physiological symptoms consist of changes associated with readiness for action. These symptoms would be adaptive if we were in fact confronting a dangerous animal. They are precisely the physiological changes necessary for fighting or fleeing. When the stress response was bred into our ancestors, the dangers they faced were short-lived. They either made their escape, killed the predator, or were eaten. Hence these physiological symptoms typically lasted only seconds or moments. Because modern stressors are mainly social or psychological, they often

**Exhibit 2–1.** Stress Model

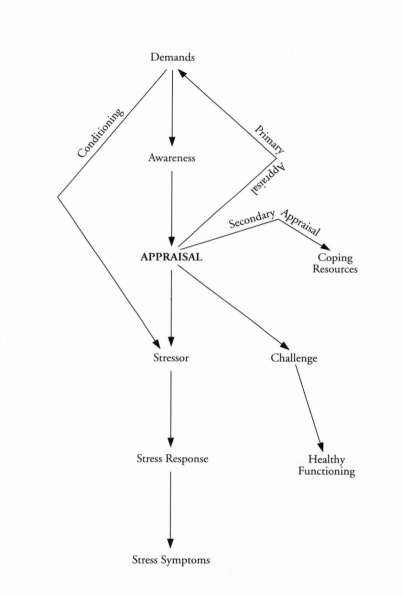

*Source:* This is a revision of a graphic constructed by K. B. Matheny, D. W. Aycock, J. L. Pugh, W. L. Curlette, and K. S. Cannella. Permission granted.

persist for days, weeks, or months and bring on psychophysiological disorders such as headaches, backaches, hypertension, and ulcers.

Behavioral symptoms include sleeplessness, restlessness, avoidance of challenging situations, tremors, and speech disturbances. Psychological symptoms of stress include increases in irritability and anxiety and difficulties with attention, perception, memory, and concentration. Physiological, behavioral, and psychological symptoms of stress interfere with work performance, are interruptive of smooth interpersonal relationships, and constitute a threat to one's health.

## The Importance of Perceived Control

Whether life's demands prove to be stressors or not depends on our perception of the adequacy of our resources for dealing with them. When demands seem serious and our resources inadequate, we conclude that the situation is out of control. Studies in psychoneuroimmunology suggest that being subjected to *un*controllable stressors suppresses immune functioning. Typical of such studies is one reported by Steven Locke wherein cancer cells injected into rats exposed to uncontrollable shocks produced tumors twice as often as in rats that could control the shocks.[4]

Similarly, Seligman, Maier, and Greer found that implanted tumors grew more rapidly and were less often rejected in animals exposed to *un*controllable stressors than in animals exposed to controllable stressors.[5] T-cells, major immune bodies, from rats exposed to controllable shock multiplied as readily as did those from unstressed rats, whereas the T-cells from rats exposed to *un*controllable shocks only multiplied weakly. Moreover, the natural killer cells (NK-cells) of rats exposed to uncontrollable shocks were less able to kill tumor cells.

Seligman, Maier, and Solomon showed that animals exposed to chronic *un*controllable stressors long enough to develop learned helplessness show a variety of disturbances when later confronted with stressors that *can* be controlled.[6] Moreover, they behave passively when confronting future stressors whether uncontrollable *or* controllable.

For twenty years Seligman has been studying the effects of uncontrollable stressors on animals and people and is convinced that helplessness is a learned reaction. As mentioned previously, when dogs trained in helplessness are later subjected to shock from which it is possible to escape, they merely lie down and whine. Seligman is convinced that people also develop learned helplessness if exposed chronically to stressful conditions over which they have no control. They no longer attempt to cope with the challenges and problems of the environment because they have come to believe that nothing they do makes any difference. The lassitude of these dogs trained in helplessness seems curiously similar to the lethargic reaction of NK-cells in confronting tumor cells on the part of rats exposed to uncontrollable stressors. It is as though the NK-cells also have lost faith in their ability to make a difference!

Jay M. Weiss observed that animals do not develop ulcers, depressed appetite, sleep disturbances, or brain-chemistry changes so characteristic of chronic stress responses if they have control over the unpleasant stimuli. It appears that the perception of control, *even when not supported by the facts*, will reduce the noxious effects of stress.[7] David Glass and Jerome Singer showed that persons exposed to loud noises while performing mental tasks later made more errors in proofreading than a second group similarly exposed but who were told that they could turn off the noise by pressing a button (even though the button did *not* actually control the noise!).[8] It appears that this principle must be well known to traffic departments that place at busy intersections buttons which supposedly will stop the traffic for pedestrians!

## Lowering Immune Defenses

Chronically experienced stress is known to lower the efficiency of the body's defense against infections and cancer. The critical element is the *extended* nature of the experience. The immunological factors affected by stress take days or weeks to change significantly. The damage to the immune system is determined more by the duration of the stressor than by its intensity. Thus, if the stressor is of sufficient duration, lymphocyte subpopulations may be significantly reduced. The following are representative studies demonstrating the weakening influence of stress on the immune system.

Janice Kiecolt-Glaser and her colleagues at the Ohio State University College of Medicine measured the effects of stress from final examinations on the immune systems of medical students.[9] They checked the NK cell count and mood states of these students one month before final exams and on the first day of exam week. Students who reported high stress from these exams had fewer active NK cells. Moreover, students who said they felt extremely lonely registered the greatest impairment to their immune systems. Results suggested that even minor stressors, such as these exams, could have a marked effect on the immune system.

Studies of marital stress clearly show the effects of stress on immune functioning. Marital disruption, either through death or divorce, is the single most powerful sociodemographic predictor of physical and emotional illness.[10] Divorce or the death of one's spouse is associated with higher rates of both infectious diseases and cancer—diseases dependent upon immune weakness.[11]

Stress from bereavement also seems to lower immune efficiency. Important immunological factors multiplied less rapidly when challenged by mitogens in bereaved spouses several weeks after the death of their spouse than in their nonbereaved counterparts.[12] Men whose wives were dying of cancer showed poorer immune functioning after the wife's death than before.[13] Moreover, even unhappiness in marriage is associated with immune suppression. In fact, in one study unhappily married partners reported poorer health than either divorced or happily married individuals of the same sex, age, and race.[14]

# Countering Conditioned Arousal

Emotional arousal from phobias or other forms of conditioning is immediate and strong, and efforts to lower it through thought control often prove ineffective. In Exhibit 2–1 notice the arrow, labeled "conditioning," which bypasses awareness and appraisal and goes directly to the stressor. Such conditioning reflects primitive nervous system wiring, which evolved to produce instantaneous reactions to acute physical dangers. Normally, neural signals are sent first from the thalamus to the cerebral cortex for appraisal; then, if appropriate, the cortex incites the emotional brain to arouse the organism to action. When confronted by threatening stimuli, however, the thalamus first stimulates the emotional brain for its immediate reaction *before* notifying the higher thought processes of the cortex. Exhibit 2–2 graphically depicts the routing of signals involved in conditioned emotional responses.

The cortex is constantly bombarded by millions of neural signals per second. If the brain responded to each of these neural signals, the result would be maddening. The reticular activating system (RAS), a way station for neural signals en route to the thalamus, serves as a reducing valve to severely limit the number of signals gaining the attention of the brain. (We will hereafter refer to signals from the RAS to the thalamus and on to the cortex as *upstream neural activity*.) Incoming signals having special significance for the person are "red flagged" by the RAS. These flagged signals are energized further by the RAS and sent on to the thalamus from where they are projected to the appropriate part of

**Exhibit 2–2.** Effects of Conditioning and Cognition on Stressful Arousal

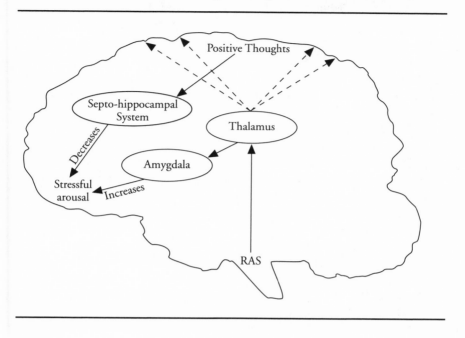

the cortex for decoding. All other signals fall coldly on the cortex without attracting its attention.

When the flagged signals reach the thalamus, they cause it to take two separate actions: it innervates the cortex in the region to which it is sending the flagged signal to insure conscious attention, and it stimulates the amygdala, a part of the emotional brain, causing it to initiate strong emotional arousal. Note that the thalamus stimulates the amygdala *before* the signal reaches the cortex for conscious appraisal. This means we often become emotionally aroused before becoming consciously aware of the threatening event. This short-circuiting of incoming signals around the conscious centers, coupled with the immediacy of emotional arousal, undoubtedly had great survival value when split-second responding made the difference between escaping and being eaten by wild animals. Under such circumstances it was functional to respond first and think later!

The immediacy of conditioned emotional responses limits the conscious control of our emotions. These responses, after all, occur before the threatening information reaches consciousness. Therefore, at times we are fated to become aroused before we can rationally appraise the seriousness of the event.

We are not totally helpless to effect our arousal from upstream neural activity, however. In Exhibit 1–3 (chapter 1) the power of thoughts to influence emotional responses (hereafter referred to as *downstream activity*) was depicted. The exhibit shows how neurons comprising positive thoughts travel downstream to the septo-hippocampal system to counter amygdala activation. If the amount of neurotransmission reaching the septo-hippocampal system exceeds that reaching the amygdala, the stressful emotional arousal will be diminished. This would seem to suggest that positive thoughts are all that are needed to lower emotional arousal. Alas, however, there is a further piece of neurological information that makes such beneficial control less automatic. The rate of neurotransmission from upstream signaling is many times greater than that from downstream signaling. It seems that nature is much more invested in our physical survival than in our happiness, and to assist survival it causes alarm signals to the amygdala to be especially powerful. Does this suggest, then, that positive thinking is worthless when competing with the stronger signals associated with emotional conditioning? Not so, for there is yet another feature of neurological functioning that must be considered.

While upstream signals are carried by high-intensity neurotransmission, the intensity of these signals steadily diminishes with time. Thus, the influence of weaker downstream signals on emotional arousal becomes relatively greater as the initial shock to the nervous system from conditioned stimuli wears off. Accordingly, there is much value in positive thinking, for it can greatly shorten the time involved in recovering from conditioned arousal.

This hopeful picture is based on the assumption that the person suffering the painful emotional arousal will respond with positive thoughts. Unfortunately, most persons actually heighten their arousal further by negative thinking. They often exaggerate the seriousness of the demand and underestimate their resources for dealing with it. Because stress is a result of perceiving that one's resources are inadequate for the demands being confronted, such thinking further strengthens the effects of upstream signals and maintains painful arousal for a much longer period.

## Active Coping Less Costly

The effects of active coping on a person's physical and mental health are quite different from the effects of passive coping. Active coping refers to efforts to eliminate the stressor or to reduce its hurtful effects. It represents adaptive coping in challenging situations, although at extreme levels it may be related to cardiovascular pathology. Passive coping, on the other hand, is associated with hypervigilance, withdrawal, and feelings of helplessness.[15]

Michael Antoni points out that the physiological pathways involved in these two ways of coping are different.[16] Active coping primarily involves activation of the SAM system (sympathetic nervous system and the adrenal medulla), which in turn releases norepinephrine and epinephrine to prepare the individual for "fight or flight." Passive coping, on the other hand, involves the HPAC system (hypothalamus, pituitary gland, and the adrenal cortices), which produces corticosteroids such as cortisol. Cortisol is known to lower immune defense and in this way to render the person more vulnerable to infectious diseases and cancer. Additionally, the helplessness associated with passive coping has been related to mental depression, and—not surprisingly—depressives are known to have a higher incidence of cancer than nondepressives. Elevations in cortisol occur in highly stressful situations in which active coping responses do *not* seem possible.

Here again perception is seen to interact with stressful life events in determining the extent of damage to the person. Perceptual patterns that typically exaggerate the seriousness of demands and minimize coping resources are very likely to lead to the overuse of passive coping with its threat to mental and physical health. Research from psychoneuroimmunology points up the paper-thin interface between the body and the mind and suggests that healthy attitudes play a powerful role in strengthening the body's natural defenses.

## Successful Coping Increases Resistance to Stress

Stress is not all bad news, however. While highly demanding life conditions may be hurtful to some, they may be *helpful to others*! Harvard researcher Steven Locke studied a group of undergraduates to determine the effect of stressful life events on the vigorousness of their immune systems.[17] He measured life events with an adaptation of the Holmes-Rahe scale and immune defense with a measure of the number and activity of NK (natural killer) cells, which are efficient in fighting cancer and viruses. In addition, he surveyed these students for signs of anxiety or depression. Students reporting high levels of anxiety or depression were considered "poor copers," and those reporting little or no anxiety or depression as "good copers."

Locke found distinct differences between the vitality of NK cells in good and poor copers. The poor copers showed the lowest NK cell activity, thus indicating greater vulnerability to cancer and infectious diseases. Surprising was the discovery that good copers showed higher NK cell activity than students who experienced *few* life demands and reported *low* levels of anxiety and depression!

Locke's research seems quite compatible with Antoni's analysis of the differential effects of SAM- and HPAC-mediated stress responses on immune functioning. Harvard students who were "good copers" and who experienced a strengthening of their immune defenses quite likely perceived the demands to be within their control and quite likely coped actively with them. Their arousal, if any, would have been triggered by the SAM system which does *not* appear to lower immune functioning. Consequently, they experienced no lowering of their NK-cell count. The "poor copers," reporting anxiety or depression in the face of high demands, quite likely perceived these demands to be beyond their control and likely adopted passive coping modes. Their arousal, on the other hand, probably was triggered by the HPAC system and led to a lowering of immune defense.

Both Antoni's analysis and Locke's research are compatible with the research of Kenneth Matheny and Penny Cupp, who found *no* relationship between life changes and subsequent illness for subjects who perceived these changes to be under their control.[18] Albert Bandura came to the same conclusion when he suggested that personal efficacy (a sense of control or mastery) is the single most effective buffer against the hurtful effects of stress.[19]

In summary, it appears that stress has a watershed effect on immune defenses. It lowers defenses in persons experiencing anxiety or depression (quite likely from perceiving demands to be *beyond* their control) and raises defenses in persons who report neither anxiety nor depression (quite likely from perceiving demands to be *within* their control).

# The Nature of the Stress Response

In order to properly understand the meaning of the physiological changes that accompany the stress response, remember that its purpose is to prepare the organism for fight or flight. While the specific effects of stressors differ significantly, their nonspecific effects are mostly the same. The organism's predictable, nonspecific reaction to stress is what Selye called the General Adaptation Syndrome (GAS).[20] This syndrome is the organism's typical manner of dealing with demands. It includes three stages: alarm, resistance, and exhaustion.

## The General Adaptation Syndrome

It might help to understand the GAS if we liken the syndrome to the reaction of a nation under attack. If at this moment a community siren sounded and we were told the country was being invaded, we would be thrust suddenly into a state of alarm. We would suspend our normal duties and gather in the squares for mutual support and direction. This state of alarm actually makes us *less* secure temporarily, since chaos would reign. Workers would leave their jobs, traffic police might leave their posts, reserves would scramble hurriedly to command centers, and many normal functions important to the survival of community life would be suspended temporarily. The community's resources would be mobilized for action once an appropriate course of action was determined.

*Alarm Stage*. Similarly, when a stressor attacks us personally, the nervous system signals a general alarm. While the process is not understood fully, it is clear that the hypothalamus (the master gland of the body buried deep within the brain), the pituitary gland (located in the same general area), and the adrenal glands (located on the tips of the kidneys) are vitally involved. The sensory input indicating danger is translated into an electrochemical signal that is carried along the afferent nervous system to the cerebral cortex, a kind of executive in charge of the organism's response. The signal is then compared with internally generated signals (memories) and interpreted in the light of these memories.

This worked-over signal is transmitted to the hypothalamus, which mobilizes emotions and muscles for appropriate action. The hypothalamus performs this vital function with the aid of the pituitary and adrenal glands. The hypothalamus stimulates the pituitary to produce adrenocorticotrophic hormone (ACTH), which, in turn, stimulates the adrenal glands to produce certain corticoids. The resulting internal reaction to these hormones in preparing the body for action is swift and predictable.

The pupils dilate to increase peripheral vision, thus allowing us to spot any blow coming from our right or left. The body's energy reserves are increased. Energy is produced by an admixture of oxygen and blood sugar; consequently, our breathing becomes faster and deeper to increase our supply of oxygen, and blood sugar levels are elevated by the liver's action in converting glycogen into glucose. The heart rate increases to speed the delivery of energy to voluntary muscles and brain. The kidneys produce vasoconstrictors, and the pituitary gland produces antidiuretic hormones to increase blood volume. The combined action of the increased heart rate. the production of vasoconstrictors, and the increased blood volume contributes to elevated blood pressure. The muscles contract to prepare for exertion. Blood is routed away from the stomach and intestines to the striated muscles to allow for a more vigorous reaction. Blood is also routed deeper, away from the skin, to prevent excessive bleeding if one is bitten or torn.

These physiological changes do little harm if they are infrequent and of short duration. However, the number of disease conditions believed to be caused, or at least worsened, by the chronic elicitation of the stress response are legend. The following examples will give the reader a fair sampling. Elevated heart rates and increased vasoconstriction may contribute to hypertension. Free fatty acids (cholesterol and triglycerides) are released into the blood stream during stressful encounters and contribute to atherosclerosis (a gradual build up of cholesterol molecules along the lining of the arteries). This condition is often the prelude to heart attacks and strokes. Cortisol, a strong stress hormone produced by the adrenal glands, suppresses the immune system. Elevated blood sugar levels may raise the set point for glucose in the hypothalamus and bring on Type II diabetes. Contracted muscles may pinch nerve endings and blood vessels, producing headaches, backaches, urinary difficulties, and other painful conditions. Elevated hydrochloric acid levels in the gastrointestinal tract increase the chances of ulcers. Sympathetic activation may cause abnormally fast heartbeats (tachycardia), a skipping of heartbeats (premature ventricular or atrial contractions), and sexual difficulties. The rerouting of the blood away from the stomach and intestines may contribute to indigestion and constipation. Constricted blood vessels may bring on migraine headaches. And poor circulation of blood to the skin may aggravate skin disorders.

*Resistance Stage*. The alarm stage is followed by the stage of resistance. In our example of a nation under siege, once the military implications of the threat have been properly assessed, appropriate forces are dispatched to combat the attackers. Resistance is then established. Similarly, the body duly assesses the perceived threat and assigns the task of resistance to certain organ systems. If the resistance is appropriate, the other systems of the body return to near normal conditions, and eventually the stressor is eliminated. This resistance is expensive, however, in terms of the amount of adaptive energy required to deal with the stressor. While the point is debatable, Selye maintains that our adaptive energy is limited by our heredity. Thus, the wasteful use of this energy through mismanaged stressors is believed to hasten the aging process.

*Exhaustion Stage.* The body's first resistance may prove inadequate to stop the invasion, and the third stage, exhaustion, is initiated. Now the body recycles into alarm until a second system for defense is activated. If the stressor persists until all adaptive energy is depleted, exhaustion then leads to death.

Although persons seem to bounce back after a bout with illness, excessive worry, depression, or some other stressor, Selye maintains that such persons are never quite the same again because some small amount of their limited adaptation energy has been used up.[21] According to Selye, this energy is stored in both a temporary tank and a reserve tank. After a bout with stressors people often *seem* as well as ever because the temporary storage tank by then has been replenished from the dwindling supply in the reserve tank. They may feel full of energy again, but the limited supply in the reserve tank now holds less than it did. In a very graphic way aging, according to Selye, can be seen as a fuel gauge for the remaining supply of reserve energy.

According to Selye, stress leaves a residue of metabolic debris that clogs up the machinery of the body and interferes with its functioning. Aging is related to this clogging—the greater the clogging, the faster the aging process. This metabolic debris takes three major forms. There are the insoluble pigments that accumulate in certain cells, such as those in the liver and the heart. There are the calcium deposits in the joints and arteries, and there is the rigidification of elastic connective tissue as a probable result of the accumulation of stable waste products that form cross-linkages between these tissues. This clogging and binding places increasing strain upon normal functioning. With enough of this metabolic debris, death becomes a certainty.

# Sources of Stress

Events and situations are not stressful in and of themselves. They become stressful only because we perceive them to exceed our resources for coping. However, there are certain factors that render us *more* likely to respond stressfully. Three such factors are (a) major life events, (b) personality variables, and (c) work conditions.

## Major Life Events

Early in this century a practicing psychiatrist, Adolph Meyer, noted a connection between the clustering of life demands and illnesses experienced by his patients.[22] He systematically gathered information regarding changes in his patients' life situations, their emotional responses to those changes, and the diseases they suffered. The results were striking. In general, the greater the life changes the greater the number and seriousness of illnesses experienced.

Hawkins, Davies, and Holmes constructed a list of life changes which commonly occurred prior to the onset of tuberculosis, cardiac disease, skin disorders, hernias, and pregnancy.[23] This list became the basis for the construction of the Schedule of Recent Experience (SRE).[24] In an attempt to add precision to the measurement of these events, survey techniques were used to establish magnitude estimates for the amount of change and readjustment associated with each life event. The form of the SRE which contains these estimated values is called the Social Readjustment Rating Scale (SRRS) and is presented in Exhibit 2–3.

Life Change Units (LCU) represent the averaged estimates by hundreds of people of the severity of the adjustment necessary to cope with each event. Marriage was arbitrarily assigned a rating of 50 LCU, and persons interviewed were asked to rate all other events in comparison with marriage. For example, the death of a spouse was believed to be twice as stressful as marriage, and so it was given a LCU of 100; a change in living conditions, on the other hand, was viewed as half as stressful, and so it was given a LCU of 25.

Thomas Holmes and Richard Rahe suggest that the risk of illness can be estimated from the magnitude of the person's LCU scores. Their simple guide suggests that a score of less than 150 LCU results in a 30 percent chance of a serious health problem in the next two years, a score between 150 and 299 LCU a 50 percent chance, and a score of 300 + an 80 percent chance.[25]

There is no doubt that many of these life demands tax one's coping resources severely. It is known, for example, that in the first year after the death of a spouse, the death rate of the remaining spouse is several times higher than that for other persons of the same age, and in the first year following divorce, persons have an illness rate twelve times greater than that of married persons.[26]

While LCU scores are related to future illness, the correlation is not strong. Rabkin and Streuning reported that correlations in most studies were around .30.[27] Although the correlation is statistically significant, the practical significance of a correlation of this magnitude is questionable since only 9 percent of the variance in illness is accounted for by LCU scores. This modest correlation quite likely reflects the failure of the instrument to take into consideration the respondent's private views of the seriousness of these life changes.

Matheny and Cupp examined the relationship between LCU scores and illness when the respondent's perception of these events *were* considered.[28] In particular, respondents were asked whether they had felt control over the event experienced, whether they had anticipated it, and whether they saw the event as being desirable. Each of these perceptions significantly lessened the relationship between these life events and subsequent illness.

Studies reviewed earlier in this chapter point to the importance of a sense of control in preventing illness when confronting stressors. Anticipating an upcoming life change allows one to marshall appropriate resources and plan strategies for dealing with it. Unanticipated change takes us off guard and often has shocking effects, like the shock that comes in stepping off a curb without knowing it is there. It seems equally likely that desirable events will be less hurtful than undesirable ones. For example, it is a good bet that the spouse seeking a divorce will suffer less from the proceedings than a spouse dragged kicking and screaming through the ordeal.

While all three of these perceptions significantly lessened the relationship between life events and illness, *control* was clearly the most important. If one felt control over experienced life events, there was no correlation between them and future illness. The message is clear: *Maintain a sense of control over life events, and they will not make you sick.*

There were clear gender differences in the life events and illness relationship. This relationship was significantly greater for women than for men. Without considering the effects of the three moderator variables (control, anticipation, and desirability), the baseline correlation was .41 for women and only .14 for men. In addition, perceived control reduced the relationship more for women than for men. This finding

**Exhibit 2-3.** Social Readjustment Rating Scale (SRRS)

| | Life Event | Life Change Units |
|---|---|---|
| 1. | Death of spouse | 100 |
| 2. | Divorce | 73 |
| 3. | Marital separation | 65 |
| 4. | Detention in jail | 63 |
| 5. | Death of close family member— (other than spouse) | 63 |
| 6. | Major personal injury or illness | 53 |
| 7. | Marriage | 50 |
| 8. | Being fired from work | 47 |
| 9. | Marital reconciliation with mate | 45 |
| 10. | Retirement from work | 45 |
| 11. | Major change in health or behavior of a family member | 44 |
| 12. | Pregnancy | 40 |
| 13. | Sexual difficulties | 39 |
| 14. | Gaining a new family member (e.g., through birth, adoption, oldster moving in, etc.) | 39 |
| 15. | Major business readjustment (e.g., merger, reorganization, bankruptcy, etc.) | 39 |
| 16. | A major change of financial state (e.g., a lot worse off or a lot better off than usual) | 38 |
| 17. | Death of close friend | 37 |
| 18. | Changing to a different line of work | 36 |
| 19. | A major change in number of arguments with spouse (e.g., either a lot more or a lot less than usual regarding child-rearing, personal habits, etc) | 36 |
| 20. | Taking out a mortgage for a major purchase (e.g., purchasing a home, business, etc.) | 31 |
| 21. | Foreclosure of mortgage or loan | 30 |
| 22. | Major change in responsibilities at work (e.g., promotion, demotion, lateral transfer) | 29 |
| 23. | Son or daughter leaving home (e.g., marriage, attending college, etc.) | 29 |
| 24. | Trouble with in-laws | 29 |
| 25. | Outstanding personal achievement | 28 |
| 26. | Wife beginning or ceasing work outside the home | 26 |
| 27. | Beginning or ceasing formal schooling | 26 |
| 28. | Major change in living conditions (e.g., building a new home, remodeling, deterioration of home or neighborhood) | 25 |
| 29. | A revision of personal habits (dress, manners, associations) | 24 |

*(Continued on next page)*

Exhibit 2-3. (Continued)

| | Life Event | Life Change Units |
|---|---|---|
| 30. | A lot more or less trouble with the boss | 23 |
| 31. | A major change in working hours or conditions | 20 |
| 32. | Change in residence | 20 |
| 33. | Changing to a new school | 20 |
| 34. | A major change in your usual type or amount of recreation | 19 |
| 35. | A major change in church activities (e.g., a lot more or less) | 19 |
| 36. | A major change in your social activities (e.g., clubs, dancing, movies, visiting) | 18 |
| 37. | Taking out a mortgage or loan for a lesser purchase | 17 |
| 38. | A major change in sleeping habits (e.g., sleeping a lot more or less, or change in part of day when asleep) | 16 |
| 39. | A major change in number of family get-togethers (e.g., a lot more or less) | 15 |
| 40. | A major change in eating habits (A lot more or less food intake, or very different meal hours or surroundings) | 15 |
| 41. | Vacation | 13 |
| 42. | Minor violations of the law (e.g., traffic tickets, jay-walking, disturbing the peace) | 11 |

*Source:* T. H. Holmes and R. H. Rahe, "The Social Adjustment Rating Scale," *Journal of Psychosomatic Research,* 11 (1967): 213–18. With permission of the exclusive license for Pergamon Microforms International Marketing Corp.

may be a result of cultural conditions that offer a greater degree of control to men than to women. In numerous surveys, women consistently report feeling less control over their lives than do men. Thus, the need for control may be more fully met (and therefore less motivating) for men than for women. If women perceive themselves as having less control than men, this may help explain the survey results of the Health Insurance Association of America that showed that women seek and get more medical services than do men.[29] More life events would be perceived as out of their control, and uncontrollable events are more likely to bring on illness.

While the relationship between desirable events and future illness was virtually zero for men (−.05), the correlation for women was a surprising .30. A similar finding was reported by Kanner and associates.[30] They compared predictions of future illness for men and women based on their hassles scores on the Hassles and Uplifts instrument. Not surprisingly, they found hassles to be related to ill health for both genders. What was surprising, however, was that *uplifts* were related to *ill* health for women!

It may be that the genders experience "desirable" events differently. Life events such as marriage, the birth of a child, and holidays are often viewed by both men and women as being desirable. The negative aspects of these "happy" events are not shared equally by men and women, however. In such experiences the woman has many more onerous responsibilities: for example, arranging the marriage, carrying and giving birth to the baby, and preparing the holiday meals. It is perhaps these taxing responsibilities accompanying otherwise desirable events that predisposes the woman to future illness.

Brown and McGill found that positive life events were detrimental to health only for persons with *low self-esteem*.[31] For persons with high self-esteem, positive events were linked to improved health. Studies such as those reported by Matheny and Cupp, Kanner and associates, and Brown and McGill demonstrate the interaction of perceptions and life events in determining illness.

## Stress-inducing Personalities

Hippocrates, the father of modern medicine, wrote, "There is no illness apart from the mind," and an ancient English physician, Parry of Bath, maintained that in caring for patients "it is much more important to know what sort of person has a disease than what sort of disease a person has." Sir William Osler, a famous Canadian physician around the turn-of-the-century, once remarked, "The care of tuberculosis depends more on what the patient has in his head than what he has in his chest." It has been suspected for centuries that the patient's attitudes and personality characteristics are very much related to the onset, course, and duration of illness. Cardiac surgeons at Rochester Medical center found that adjusted patients survived heart bypass operations ten times better than depressed ones. Depression, of course, is associated with chronic stress.

*The Anxious Reactive Personality.* Daniel Girdano and George Everly maintain that certain persons overreact to fearful and frustrating experiences and, consequently, are likely to experience a great deal more stress than persons less prone to overreact.[32] Three patterns of physiological response can be seen among persons confronting fearful stimuli. With Pattern A, the normal response, arousal increases sharply upon the appearance of a fearful stimulus, but it gradually diminishes. With Pattern B, the pattern of meditators, arousal also increases sharply, but it falls off much more rapidly than for normals.[33] With Pattern C, the response of the anxious reactive personality, arousal increases as with the other patterns, but it continues to feed on itself and in this way increases for some time.

Girdano and Everly explained that anxious reactive personalities initially react to the fearful stimulus in the normal manner, but then their arousal soars as they react anxiously to their own symptoms. The sensations associated with anxiety become cues to further trigger stress reactivity. Thus a positive feedback loop results wherein anxiety feeds on itself.

Anxious reactive persons catastrophize, that is they greatly magnify potential dangers in their lives. Monte Buchsbaum referred to such persons as "augmenters," persons who have a natural tendency to exaggerate the threat posed by a given situation. Persons with the opposite perceptual tendencies were said to be "reducers."[34]

Anxious reactive persons appear to relive the same fearful situation for days or weeks after the incident is over. They are aroused by some undesirable situation. They further heighten arousal by catastrophizing. After some time, the arousal begins to wear off, but they mentally rehearse the unpleasant scene, and the symptoms return.

*Coronary Prone Personality*. Much has been written about the coronary prone personality with its Type A behavior pattern. According to the discoverers of this personality type, Meyer Friedman and Ray Rosenman, coronary prone individuals suffer from "hurry sickness," that is from the need to do more and more in less and less time.[35] Type A individuals are constantly racing the clock in an effort to produce. The cardinal dynamic underlying their behavioral pattern is the conviction that they are not natively worth much, *that their value comes solely from their productions*. Consequently, when they are not getting things done, they begin to feel worthless. In order to avoid feelings of worthlessness, they maintain a constant backlog of tasks and fill every hour with activity.

Friedman and Rosenman define the Type A behavior pattern as "an action-emotion complex that can be observed in any person who is aggressively involved in a chronic, incessant struggle to achieve more and more in less and less time, and, if required to, does so against the opposing efforts of other things or persons."[36] Because they try to do more than others, and to do it in less time, they are particularly vulnerable to frustration. Because frustration leads naturally to hostility, Type A individuals experience more hostility than others. Their Type A characteristics — competitiveness, impatience, and aggressiveness — keep them in a chronic state of sympathetic nervous system arousal. According to Friedman and Rosenman, Type A persons suffer 66 percent more heart attacks than their Type B counterparts. A partial list of Type A symptoms is presented in Exhibit 2–4.

Although there is no formal scoring key for this list, you are likely to be a Type A if you answered "yes" to five or more of these questions. Friedman and Rosenman estimate that 60 percent of Americans have Type A patterns. Modern stress researchers, however, acknowledge up to six different subpatterns representing differing degrees of Type A characteristics.

David McClelland discovered a correlation between highly promotable managers and Type A characteristics.[37] His promotable managers had a high need for power, a low need for establishing friendly relations with others—affiliation, and a high need for self-control, inhibition. Moreover, he found that these managers were more frequently ill than

**Exhibit 2–4.** Symptoms of Type A Behavior

1. Do you have a habit of explosively accentuating key words in your ordinary speech and finishing your sentences in a burst of speed?
2. Do you *always* move, walk, and eat rapidly?
3. Do you feel (and openly show) impatience with the rate at which most events take place? Do you find it difficult to restrain yourself from hurrying the speech of others?
4. Do you get unduly irritated at delay—when the car in front of you seems to slow you up, when you have to wait in line, or wait to be seated in a restaurant?
5. Does it bother you to watch someone else perform a task you know you can do faster?
6. Do you often try to do two things at once (dictate while driving or read business papers while you eat)?
7. Do you *always* find it difficult to refrain from talking about or bringing the themes of any conversation around to those subjects that interest you, and when unable to, do you merely pretend to listen?
8. Do you almost always feel vaguely guilty when you relax and do absolutely nothing for several hours to several days?
9. Are you so preoccupied that you fail to observe important or lovely objects in your environment?
10. Do you leave little or no time to become things worth *being* because you are so busy getting things worth *having*?

From *Type A Behavior and Your Heart* by M. Friedman and R. Rosenman (New York: Knopf, 1974), copyright 1974 by Meyer Friedman. Reprinted by permission of Alfred A. Knopf, Inc.

were managers with lesser power needs but greater needs for affiliation or managers with high power needs but lower needs for inhibition.

Type A individuals with charismatic qualities, however, may actually be healthier than mellower Type B's. Even though these charismatic types are just as speedy, driven, and ambitious as other Type A's, they are more emotionally expressive, and less hostile — probably because they are more effective in enlisting the help of others. They laugh infectiously, move a lot, and appear to be genuinely confident. As a result they are less prone to heart disease.

It now seems that only part of the Type A pattern may be coronary prone. According to Redford Williams and his colleagues at Duke University, the toxic part appears to be hostility associated with "cynical contempt."[38] Such persons are deeply suspicious and constantly on guard against others whom they believe are dishonest, antisocial, and immoral. The Duke team found that lawyers having high scores on a hostility scale were four times more likely to die by age fifty than men who had low hostility scores. They concluded that this type of hostility predicts death, not only from blockages to the coronary arteries but from other causes as well. A similar outcome was reported by Dembroski and associates.[39] They found that, among all the Type A factors, only "potential for hostility" and "anger-in," a tendency to swallow one's anger rather than to express it, were predictors of coronary artery disease. In another analysis they found these factors to be interactive, that is the potential for hostility was associated with coronary artery disease only for patients who were also high on the anger-in dimension. The lethal combination, then, appears to be:

HOSTILITY + CYNICAL DISTRUST + ANGER-IN.

This research strongly suggests the potential usefulness of assertiveness training as a buffer against heart attacks. Assertiveness should not be confused with aggressiveness. Assertiveness is the honest, straightforward expression of what one feels, believes, and wants to have happen *without trying to make others do it*! When we feel exploited and do nothing about it, we end up being angry with two people — the exploiter *and* ourselves.

The hurry sickness, polyphasic behavior, and multiple goals so characteristic of Type A persons make them more susceptible to frustration, and thus hostility, than persons not sharing these characteristics. While hostility may be the only Type A factor directly predictive of heart disease, the other Type A characteristics may indirectly contribute to the prediction by predisposing the person to increased amounts of hostility.

If, indeed, chronic hostility, swallowed or expressed, contributes to coronary artery disease, the remedy, of course, would be to avoid the hostility if possible. One may help reduce the hostility by lessening features contributing to the hurry sickness (over-ambitiousness, failure to give oneself ample time capsules in which to accomplish one's tasks, the belief that one's value derives solely from one's accomplishments, and trying to do multiple tasks at the same time).

*Disease-Prone Personality.* Friedman and Booth-Kewley conducted a meta-analysis of studies examining the relationship between personality characteristics and specific illnesses.[40] More particularly, depression, anger, and anxiety were related to asthma, arthritis, ulcers, headaches, and coronary artery disease. Except for coronary artery disease, they found little support for the assumption that specific emotional dispositions lead to specific illnesses. They did find, however, the likely existence of a generic "disease-prone personality" that involves all three of the emotions (depression, anger, and anxiety).

In recent years a great deal of attention has been directed to the role of anger/hostility in causing illness; however, the most striking single relationship evident in the Friedman and Booth-Kewley study is between *depression* and the diseases investigated (except for ulcers). The researchers surmise that these negative emotional dispositions may function like an inadequate diet that predisposes one to all sorts of diseases.

Positive attitudes leading to positive emotions appear to be powerfully therapeutic. In his best selling book, *Love Medicine and Miracles*, Bernie Siegel, M.D., writes "Happy people are not usually the ones who get sick. In fact, a positive attitude may be the single most important factor in healing or staying well."[41] The Friedman and Booth-Kewley study mentioned earlier appears to support Siegel's contention. Another study of two hundred Harvard graduates, asked to undergo physical exams every five years and to answer personality surveys every two years for fifty years, also strongly suggests that happiness immunizes one against disease. Only 3 percent of those who seemed happiest became chronically ill or died, compared with the 38 percent who seemed least happy. This was true even after alcohol, tobacco, obesity, and family history were taken into account.[42]

## Rigidly Held Belief Systems

In chapter 1, we discussed the critical importance of control for the prevention of stress. We might speculate that this powerful need for control originates from feelings of insecurity. The experience of being a passenger in an auto that is sliding on slippery roads demonstrates well the importance of feeling in control. The experience is much more frightening if we do not have *our* hands on the wheel!

The need for control creates a compulsion to "know." We cannot control events that we cannot predict, and we cannot predict accurately if we do not know how things operate. There is so much emotional satisfaction in "knowing" that we often resist information that questions the accuracy of our beliefs. The old insecurities revisit us when our sacred views are challenged. Indeed, to protect rigidly held beliefs we must often disregard our own experience. Thus, our view of reality is limited by selective perception.

The world is in a constant state of flux, and to adjust to it requires constant recalibration of our sights. Rigidly held beliefs limit our responsiveness to the changing scene. The tendency is to take a still shot of a moving target and to contend that our picture is complete and accurate. Our still shot often is inadequate in guiding our aim. Thus, we are fated to miss the target quite often. To stay on target we must change course like a ground-to-air missile. The missile is launched in the direction of the moving plane, but it must make repeated self-corrections before striking the target. We should not disregard the experience of parents, teachers, and religious leaders, but we should not discount our own experience either. If we discount our experience in favor of the authorities, we soon begin to lose self-confidence and self-respect. Some practices learned in childhood may become anachronistic, that is, they are no longer useful. They may have been appropriate at some point in time, but as conditions changed, they became less and less useful. A beautiful example of outdated teaching was the saber-toothed tiger curriculum taught West African youth for decades after the tigers had died out. When these ferocious animals had stalked their kin, such teaching had great survival value. But with the last of these animals gone from their region, the teaching was useless and wasteful. Some rules we learned as children may not serve us well as adults. Because we find great emotional satisfaction in firm beliefs, we may hold on to outdated beliefs that are no longer good guides to behavior. Efforts to meet our needs using these guidelines are likely to prove ineffective, and we are likely to suffer stress from the resulting frustration.

In summary, our insecurity leads to the need to control events, which leads to the need to predict events, which leads to the need to understand events. Knowing, then, is highly reinforcing as it greatly lessens basic insecurity. Resulting belief systems, thus, are highly resistive to change, even though they may be inadequate guides for meeting our needs and may create much stress. Our beliefs represent mere facsimiles of reality and they will require frequent updating. Consequently, we become angry when events do not go according to our beliefs. We are intolerant of behavior that does not fit our models of how things operate. We become childish, impatient, and puckish—insisting that others conform to our views of how they should behave.

A principal function of religion is to help devotees to gain new perspective on life. In order to attain this new perspective, they are given various prescriptions: to assume an innocence of perception, to view things as openly as a small child, to "be not conformed to the world but be transformed by the renewing of your minds," to view things from "big mind" rather than "small mind," to look at the world with "soft" eyes rather than "hard" eyes. Some religious systems that exhort us to rebel against inadequate ways of perceiving reality sometimes freeze this new perspective into rigid dogma—a once-and-for-all statement of how things *really* are and *really* work. When these representations of reality are accurate, they make our adjustment to reality more appropriate; when, however, they are inaccurate, our adjustment becomes more and more out of sync with reality. Like a cart with its wheels off center at the axle, we thrust and pitch forward under great strain. If these views are grossly unrepresentative of reality, they may lead to behavior that does great harm. For example, children are sometimes the victims of parental beliefs that prohibit blood transfusions or other vital medical services.

How then are we to treat our models of reality. The Harvard psychologist, Gordon Alport, suggested that we hold "tentative convictions."[43] The advice seems paradoxical; we must base our behavior on beliefs we are convinced are correct, but we are to hold them *loosely*. We are to remain open to information that challenges the accuracy of such beliefs, and when our experience contradicts them, we are to recast them into more workable models.

## Addictive Desires

Much stress and unhappiness arise from desires so compulsive that they function like addictions. When these desires are unfulfilled, we grow demanding and impatient. We become critical of others for not meeting our "needs." We make no distinction between *needs* that are necessary for our physical survival and *wants* that are unnecessary but desirable. When these terms are used properly, thirst, hunger, and rest are considered needs, whereas the desire for a new auto or for attention from others would be examples of wants.

Both needs and wants, of course, are common and motivating. Indeed, the role of advertising in a capitalist economy is to create such desires. While all desires have the potential for creating stress, they are particularly stressful when we are addicted to having them fulfilled. When addictive desires are unmet, we become intolerant and surly with others. Even if we satisfy many such addictions during the day, the one unmet addiction will prey on our consciousness and make us unhappy.

The proper strategy for preventing much stress from these insistent desires is to upgrade wants to preferences.[44] We must reframe these wants as preferable but not necessary for our happiness. We should say "I'd rather my plane would arrive on time so I can make my connec-tion," rather than "This plane's *got* to arrive on time so I can make my connection!" You hope your arrival is on time, as this is considerably more convenient, but you remind yourself that you can adjust to the temporary inconvenience if necessary. You would simply *prefer* the smoother connection. If there is a reasonable course of action that you can take to secure your preference, you will take it. If not, you will merely adjust.

Persons addicted to having their wants met believe an injustice has been done them when these needs are not met and often criticize others for their "lack of consideration." The resulting frustration causes them to pump out massive amounts of stress hormones and to cycle into a flight-fight mode. With their anger out of control, they often trigger negative reactions in others. This addictive response is not only expen-sive in terms of emotional energy, it is often counterproductive as well.

The *Pali Cannon* suggests that all human misery derives from these addictive desires. We are said to make ourselves unhappy by constantly agitating ourselves with cravings for one thing or another. A kind of inflation sets in, and we require more and more in order to be satisfied. Emerson once wrote that the pain of doing without is greater than the pleasure of possessing.[45] Thus, the more things we surround ourselves with, the more we must work to maintain the same level of satisfaction. The loss of these things is likely to cost us more inconvenience than the pleasure their possession brings.

Obviously, it is impossible to live in the world without wanting things. We would be happier, however, if we could weaken the tyranny of such desires, to learn to view them as preferences rather than essentials. But how do we temper these addictive desires? William James, America's most eminent nineteenth-century psychologist, suggested we could gain freedom from addictive desires by making them mute. He wrote: "Refuse to express an emotion, and it dies. . . . We feel sorry because we cry, angry because we strike, afraid because we tremble, and not that we cry, strike, or tremble because we are sorry, angry, or fearful."[46] He maintained that behavior creates the feelings. Thus, if we behave differently we will feel differently. This appears to be the basis for the Stanislavski method for acting. Students of the method are challenged to live the role, for then the appropriate feelings will come. We increase our selfishness by greedy behavior and, on the other hand, we may temper our selfishness by directing attention and energy to behavior that is in the public interest. The Viennese psychiatrist Alfred Adler maintained that depressed persons would be greatly improved within two weeks if they would focus their attention and energy on the welfare of others.[47]

James further suggested that because "Nature abhors a vacuum," it is helpful to try to *replace* inappropriate behaviors with more appropriate ones rather than simply to eliminate them. "If we wish to conquer undesirable emotional tendencies, we must assiduously go through the outward movements of those contrary dispositions that we prefer to cultivate."[48] This idea of replacing bad behavior with good was expressed in the New Testament parable wherein a room swept clean of devils but, left empty, was later refilled with seventy times seventy demons. If the addict is asked to give up the pleasurable habit without a satisfactory replacement, the battle is indeed a tough one. Perhaps it is for this reason that so many efforts by the public to stop substance abuse fail. Harvey Milkman and Stanley Sunderwirth suggest offering the addict socially acceptable behaviors that roughly simulate the same feeling state invoked by the addiction.[49] They maintain that we are addicted to feeling states triggered by certain rates of neurotransmission within the brain. The particular substance or activity to which one is addicted is merely an instrument to incite these feelings. They hold that it would be possible to identify a menu of nonhurtful activities that would nicely replace the prohibited substance or activity. While a full complement of such activities has not yet been constructed, they do offer us some examples in their work. The point is that you likely will be more success-ful in efforts to rid yourself of self-defeating habits if you seek to replace them with other activities that are rewarding. Be careful, however, that you do not replace one bad habit with another.

If this prescription of James and Adler for selfless behavior is taken to the extreme, it may create stress by frustrating legitimate needs and wants. Gotama, the Buddha, in his search for peace and meaning, took on the ascetic life of a Hindu sect. Much like medieval Christian monas-tic orders, the sect sought to free the spirit by denying the body. It was believed that a state of conflict existed between the spirit and the flesh and that one could strengthen the spirit by weakening the body. Gotama soon observed that efforts to deny his body of food, liquids, or rest merely trapped his attention and *obstructed* his spiritual growth. He concluded that a "middle way" between deprivation and indulgence was better. This middle way of moderation holds promise for stressless living. It suggests that one should work diligently to meet basic needs, then treat everything else as a want to be preferred but not demanded. In most approaches to life, moderation seems healthy, whereas excessiv-ity or addictiveness seems to create much stress and unhappiness. The goal for dealing with addictive desires appears fourfold:

- Carefully discriminate between *needs* that the body must have and *wants* that would merely make life more pleasant.
- Upgrade addictions to preferences — learn to say "I would *prefer* that . . . ."
- Choose a middle path between deprivation and indulgence; that is, practice moderation.
- When trying to eliminate addictions, seek to replace them with more acceptable behaviors.

A new perspective regarding one's desires is necessary. Remind yourself of the tyranny imposed by addictive wants and of the inflation that sets in when trying to satisfy them. Addictions typically require more and more for their satisfaction. What results is a life of servitude in trying to meet them.

## Stressful Working Conditions

Albert Camus wrote "Without work, all life goes rotten, but when work is soulless, life stifles and dies."[50] A World Health Organization

(WHO) report suggests that roughly 50 percent of workers are unhappy in their jobs. Approximately 75 percent of persons seeking psychiatric consultation are experiencing problems that can be traced to a lack of job satisfaction or an inability to unwind.[51] The problem is that work and the workplace have been designed almost exclusively for efficiency and cost without serious concern for the well-being of workers. The Department of Health and Human Services reports that approximately 110 million U.S. workers are exposed to occupational hazards that can pose significant risks to their health.[52] If the workplace will not clean up its act to prevent physical injury and illness, it is even less likely to be concerned with enhancing the psychological growth and well-being of workers.

For many, the workplace is a major stressor. The rash of mergers and acquisitions in the eighties is an example of the "combination stress" brought on by the turmoil and displacement that accompanies it. Such moves frequently devastate employees who may have felt a significant measure of control before the change. In one study, eleven million workers reported health-endangering levels of "mental stress" at work. Only one other hazardous work condition—loud noise—was found to be more prevalent.[53] In a study by the National Council on Compensation Insurance, claims for gradual mental stress (cumulative emotional problems that stem from psychosocial stressors at work) account for about 11 percent of all claims for occupational disease, and the costs of workers' compensation for gradual mental stress surpassed the average cost of claims for other occupational diseases.

Certain conditions in the workplace prove particularly stressful for workers. Figuring prominently among them is the feeling of being powerless to make changes necessary for the successful performance of one's duties. The organizational structure of many agencies and corporations is still military, and hence, decisions are made from the top down. Stress is sometimes defined as *responsibility without control*. Evidence is growing that control is the decisive factor in determining the health consequences of work demands—adverse effects on health occur primarily when control is not commensurate with demands.[54] Quite often managers are given broad responsibilities without the necessary resources to carry them out. They feel their authority has been emasculated, that they are required to manage employees without adequate sanctions for motivating them. Powerlessness often results from being shut out of the decision-making process. Research regarding worker participation in making decisions suggests that emotional distress, lowered self-esteem, and job dissatisfaction result from nonparticipation of workers.[55]

The Swedish Government Commission for Work Environment and Health 1990 report concluded that the work conditions most adverse to worker health are most likely to be found in the health care professions, blue-collar jobs, and the transportation industry.[56] The common denominator of these jobs is that they expose workers to a combination of high psychosocial stress, heavy work loads, and a low level of decision latitude.[57] The amount of decision latitude given workers may determine whether occupational demands will be the "spice of life" or the "kiss of death."[58]

The absence of positive feedback contributes to worker stress. Few things are more motivating than full appreciation for work done. Some managers, however, believe that praising workers is bribery, that it is inappropriate to reward workers when they are "merely doing their duty." Such managers often feel free to give negative feedback, however. Worse yet is the manager who gives *no* feedback, positive or negative. Many workers experience a complete absence of feedback as quite stressful.

Abrasive relationships with colleagues, supervisors, and subordinates at work are significant stressors.[59] Minimal opportunities to interact with other workers is a stressor for many workers.[60] We are social animals, and most persons feel deprived when they cannot engage in social exchanges with other workers. A study of over one thousand male workers showed that social support from supervisors and fellow workers buffered the stressful effects of job demands, including depression, which often result in job dissatisfaction.[61]

Workers respond differently to work conditions, but many will also find the following conditions to be stressful: repetitive, machine-paced work;[62] role conflicts resulting from the expectations of multiple supervisors;[63] role ambiguity;[64] rotating shifts;[65] career insecurity;[66] unclear decision making authority; role overload and underload; tight deadlines; constant changes in procedures, schedules, or supervision; and conditions threatening to the worker's health.

Kobassa found that certain managers experienced far less stress from their work than did others.[67] These managers were considered "hardy." Typical of these hardy workers were characteristics referred to as the Three Cs: Challenge, Commitment, and Control. Managers who found their work to be appropriately challenging, who were committed to succeed at it, and who felt they had most conditions under control appeared to be immunized against the stressful effects of work pressures. Although Kobassa's research was done on managers, hardiness with the three Cs is likely to be a significant buffer against stress for workers at all levels

Both the worker and the organization have contributions to make to worker hardiness. Management can help the worker's sense of challenge by more careful placement to insure a good match between worker interest and ability and the demands of the job. Management can make it easier for workers to feel committed to the job by providing more meaningful work through job enrichment, job enlargement, or job rotation. Fragmented, short-cycle tasks that provide little stimulation and allow little use of worker skills or creativity have little intrinsic challenge.[68] Moreover, management can strengthen the worker's sense of control by offering greater latitude for worker decisions. On the other hand, workers can improve their sense of challenge by seeking more challenging work and by raising their personal standards for performance. They can increase their commitment by reminding themselves of the importance of their work to product control and consumer satisfaction. The can contribute somewhat to their sense of control by reminding themselves of the control they do have.

In general, it can be concluded that pathogenic stress is more likely to be encountered on the job if a mismatch exists between the abilities of workers and job demands, if workers feel little control over their work conditions, if they experience little social support on the job, and if their coping resources are deficient.

# Summary

Mismanaged stress is a major cause of illness, ruptured interpersonal relationships, and work failures. Perception plays a powerful role in determining whether demands will prove to be stressors. If one perceives demands to be greater than personal resources for coping with them, the stress response is automatically triggered. The stress response consists of predictable physiological, behavioral, and psychological changes to prepare the person to deal with emergencies. Whereas such radical mobilization of resources was necessary in order for our ancestors to deal with ever-present dangers in their environment, this primordial response is clearly inappropriate for the more quiescent experiences of modern life. Consequently, our nervous systems today are wired to overrespond to any perceived threat.

Chronic stress is implicated as a causal or aggravating factor in many diseases. Some stress hormones are known to be immunosuppressive and others are believed to contribute to heart disease. At times, certain mental conditions such as depression are also thought to be caused or worsened by stress. Potential stressors include clustering life events, stress-inducing personalities (such as the coronary-prone, the anxious reactive, and the disease-prone), and certain work conditions.

## ENDNOTES

1. A. T. W. Simeons, *Man's Presumptuous Brain: An Evolutionary Interpretation of Psychosomatic Disease* (New York: E. P. Dutton, 1961).

2. Hans Selye, *The Stress of Life* (New York: McGraw Hill, 1986).

3. R. S. Lazarus and S. Folkman, *Stress, Appraisal and Coping* (New York: Springer, 1984).

4. Steven Locke, *The Healer Within* (New York: New American Library, 1986).

5. Martin Seligman, S. Maier, and J. Greer, "The Alleviation of Learned Helplessness in the Dog," *Journal of Abnormal and Social Psychology* 3 (1968): 256–262.

6. Martin Seligman, S. Maier, and R. Soloman, "Unpredictable and Uncontrollable Aversive Events," in *Aversive Conditioning and Learning*, ed. F. R. Brush (New York: Academic Press, 1971), 215.

7. Jay M. Weiss, "Ulcers," in *Psychopathology: Experimental Models*, ed. Jack Maser and Martin Seligman (San Francisco: Greeman, 1977), 22.

8. David C. Glass and Jerome Singer, *Urban Stress* (New York: Academic Press, 1972), 126.

9. Janice Kiecolt-Glasser, et al., "Psychosocial Modifiers of Immunocompetence in Medical Students," *Journal of Behavioral Medicine* 7 (1984): 1–12.

10. A. R. Somers, "Marital Status, Health, and Use of Health Services, *Journal of the American Medical Association* 241 (1979): 1818–1822.

11. V. I. Ernster, S. Selvin, and N. L. Petrakis, "Cancer Incidence by Marital Status: U.S. Third National Cancer Survey," *Journal of National Cancer Institute* 63 (1979): 585–587; J. Lynch, *The Broken Heart* (New York: Basic Books, 1977); A. R. Somers, ibid.

12. R. W. Bartrop, et al., "Depressed Lymphocyte Function After Bereavement," *Lancet* 1 (1977): 834–836; M. Irwin, M. Daniels, et al., "Impaired Natural Killer Cell Activity During Bereavement," *Brain, Behavior, and Immunity* 1 (1987): 98–104.

13. S. J. Schleifer, et al., "Suppression of Lymphocyte Stimulation Following Bereavement, *Journal of the American Medical Association* 250 (1983): 374–377.

14. K. S. Renne, "Health and Marital Experience in an Urban Population," *Journal of Marriage and the Family* 23 (1971):338–350.

15. P. McCabe and N. Schneiderman, "Psychophysiologic Reactions To Stress," in *Behavioral Medicine: The Biopsychosocial Approach*, ed. by A. N. Schneiderman and J. Tapp (New Jersey: Lawrence Erlbaum Associates, 1985).

16. Michael Antoni, "Neuroendocrine Influence in Psychoimmunology and Neoplasis: A Review," *Psychology and Health* 1, no. 1 (1987): 3–24.

17. Steven Locke, *The Healer Within* (New York: New American Library, 1986).

18. Kenneth B. Matheny and Penny Cupp, "Control, Desirability, and Anticipation As Moderating Variables Between Life Change and Illness," *Journal of Human Stress* 9 (1983):14–23.

19. Albert Bandura, "Self-efficacy Mechanism in Human Agency," *American Psychologist* 37, no. 2(1982): 137–144.

20. Hans Selye, *The Stress of Life* (New York: McGraw Hill, 1986).

21. Ibid.

22. Adolph Meyer, "The Life Chart and the Obligation of Specifying Positive Data in Psychopathological Diagnosis," in *The Collected Papers of Adolph Meyer,* vol. 3, ed. by E. Winters (Baltimore: The Johns Hopkins Press).

23. N. G. Hawkins, R. Davies, and T. H. Holmes, "Evidence of Psychosocial Factors in the Development of Pulmonary Tuberculosis," *American Review of Tuberculosis and Pulmonary Disorders* 75 (1957): 768–780.

24. Thomas Holmes and Richard Rahe, "The Social Readjustment Rating Scale," *Journal of Psychosomatic Research* 11, 213–218.

25. Ibid.

26. M. Young, B. Benjamin, and C. Wallace, "The Mortality of Widowers," *Lancet* 3, (1960): 254–256.

27. J. G. Rabkin and E. H. Struening, "Life Events, Stress, and Illnesss," *Science* 194 (1976): 1013–1020.

28. Kenneth B. Matheny and Penny Cupp, "Control."

29. Health Insurance Association of America, "Women Surpass Men in Visiting Doctors," *Health Insurance News* (Washington, D.C.: Health Insurance Association of America, 1981).

30. A. D. Kanner, et al., "Comparison of Two Models of Stress Measurement: Daily Hassles and Uplifts vs. Major Life Events," *Journal of Behavioral Medicine* 4 (1981): 1–39.

31. J. D. Brown and K. S. McGill, "The High Cost of Success: When Positive Life Events Product Negative Health Consequences." Paper delivered at annual meeting of American Psychological Association, Atlanta, Georgia, 1988.

32. Daniel Girdano and George Everly, *Controlling Stress and Tension* (Englewood Cliffs, New Jersey: Prentice-Hall, 1979).

33. Daniel Goleman, "Meditation As Metatherapy," *Journal of Transpersonal Psychology* 1 (1971): 1–25.

34. Monte S. Buchsbaum, "The Sensoristat in the Brain," *Psychology Today* (May 1978): 97–104.

35. Meyer Friedman and Ray H. Rosenman, *The Type A Behavior and Your Heart* (Greenwich, Connecticut: Fawcett Publications, 1981), 194.

36. Ibid.

37. David C. McClelland, "Sources of Stress in the Drive for Power," in *Psychopathology of Human Adaptation*, ed. George Serban (New York: Plenum Press, 1976).

38. Redford B. Williams, et al., "Type A Behavior, Hostility, and Coronary Artheroschlerosis," *Psychosomatic Medicine* 47 (1980): 539–549.

39. T. M. Dembroski, et al., "Components of Type A, Hostility, and Anger-In: Relationship to Angiographic Findings," *Psychosomatic Medicine* 47, no. 3 (1985): 219–232.

40. H. S. Friedman and S. Booth-Kewley, "The Disease-Prone Personality: A Meta-Analysis View of the Construct," *American Psychologist* 42, no. 6 (1987): 539–555.

41. Bernie S. Siegel, *Love, Medicine and Miracles* (New York: Harper & Row, 1986).

42. G. G. Vaillant, *Adaptation to Life* (Boston: Little, Brown, 1977).

43. Gordon Alport, *Becoming: Basic Considerations for a Psychology of Personality* (New Haven: Yale University Press, 1955).

44. Ken Keyes, *Handbook to Higher Consciousness* (St. Mary, Kentucky: Living Love Center), 43–47, 49.

45. Ralph Waldo Emerson, "Self Reliance" in *The World in Literature*, vol. II, ed. George Anderson and Robert Warnock (Glenview, Illinois, 1967), 559.

46. William James, *Principles of Psychology*, vol. II (New York: Dover, 1890), 87.

47. Alfred Adler, *What Life Should Mean to You* (New York: Dryden Press, 1958).

48. William James, *Principles of Psychology*, vol. II, 89.

49. Harvey Milkman and Stanley Sunderwirth, *Craving for Ecstasy* (Lexington, Massachuetts: D. C. Heath and Company, 1987).

50. Albert Camus, *The Myth of Sisyphys* (New York: Knopf, 1955), 26.

51. L. Levi, "Psychosomatic Disease as a Consequence of Occupational Stress," in *Psychosocial Factors at Work and Their Relation to Health*, ed. R. Kalimo, M.A. El-Batawi and C. L. Cooper (Geneve, Switzerland: World Health Organization, 1987), 78–91.

52. Department of Health and Human Services, *Disease Prevention/Health Promotion: The Facts* (Palo Alto, California: Bull, 1989).

53. S. Shilling, and R. M. Brackbill, "Occupational Health and Safety Risks and Potential Health Consequences Perceived by U. W. Workers," *Public Health Reports* 102 (1987): 36–46.

54. S. L. Sauter, J. J. Hurrell, Jr., and C. L. Cooper, eds., *Job Control and Worker Health* (New York: Wiley, 1989).

55. B. L. Margolis, W. H. Kroes and R. A. Quinn, "Job Stress: An Unlisted Occupational Hazard," *Journal of Occupational Medicine* 16 (1974): 654–661; P. E. Spector, "Perceived Control by Employees: A Meta-analysis of Studies Concerning Autonomy and Participation in Decision Making," *Human Relations* 39 (1986): 1005–1016.

56. Swedish Government Commission for Work Environment and Health, *Jobs Exposed to Special Health Risks* (Stockholm, Sweden: Allmanna Forlaget, 1990).

57. Robert A. Karasek and Tores Theorell, *Healthy Work: Stress, Productivity and the Reconstruction of Working Life* (New York: Basic Books, 1990).

58. L. Levi, "Occupational Stressors, Biological Stress and Workers' Health," *Journal of the University of Occupational and Environmental Health* 11 (1989): 229–245.

59. T. A. Beehr and J. E. Newman, "Job Stress, Employee Health, and Organizational Effectiveness: A Facet Analysis, Model, and Literature Review," *Personnel Psychology* 31 (1978): 665–669.

60. S. Cobb and S. V. Kasl, *Termination: The Consequences of Job Loss*, DHEW NIOSH Publication No.77–1261 (Washington, D. C.: U.S. Government Printing Office, 1977).

61. R. A. Karasek, J. Schwartz and T. Theorell, *Job Characteristics, Occupation, and Coronary Heart Disease* (Final report on Grant No. R-01-OH00906). (Cincinnati, Ohio: National Institute for Occupational Safety and Health, 1982).

62. J. J. Hurrell, Jr., and M. M. Colligan, "Machine-pacing and Shiftwork: Evidence for Job Stress," *Journal of Organizational Behavior Management* 8 (1987): 159–175.

63. S. Jackson and R. Schuler, "A Meta-analysis and Conceptual Critique of Research on Role Ambiguity and Role Conflict in Work Settings," *Organizational Behavior and Human Decisions* 36 (1985): 16–28.

64. R. L. Kahn, et al., *Organizational Stress: Studies in Role Conflict and Ambiguity* (New York: Wiley, 1964).

65. L. C. Johnson, et al., eds., *The Twenty-four Hour Workday: Proceedings of a Symposium on Variations in Work-sleep Schedules* (DHHS Publication No. 81–127). (Washington, D. C.: U.S. Government Printing Office).

66. V. J. Sutherland and C. L. Cooper, "Sources of Work Stress," in *Occupational Stress: Issues and Developments in Research*, ed. J. J. Hurrell, et al. (London: Taylor & Francis, 1988), 3–39.

67. S. Kobassa, "Stressful Life Events, Personality, and Health: An Inquiry Into Hardiness," *Journal of Personality and Social Psychology* 37 (1979): 1–11.

68. T. Cox, "Repetitive Work: Occupational Stress and Health," in *Job Stress and Blue Collar Work*, ed. C. L. Cooper and M. Smith (London: Wiley, 1985), 85–112.

# PREVENTING STRESS BUILDUP

The mind is its own place, and one can make a heaven of hell,
a hell of heaven.

——John Milton

The last chapter was devoted to an understanding of the nature, sources, and effects of stress. Comprehensive approaches to coping include efforts to prevent stress and efforts to combat it effectively once it is initiated. This chapter offers promising ways of preventing stress, and chapter 4 will present strategies for combating stressors once they have been encountered.

Preventive coping includes efforts to strengthen the body's general resistance to stress, to alter stress-inducing behavior patterns, to avoid unnecessary stressors, to develop a sense of control over events in one's life, to build additional resources for coping, and to achieve a more serene state of consciousness. Effective efforts at prevention will significantly decrease the need for combative coping. Therefore, most of the work should be done at the preventive level. Benjamin Franklin's adage, "An ounce of prevention is worth a pound of cure," is certainly true in this case.

# Strengthen General Resistance to Stress

One's reaction to stressors is influenced significantly by one's health and fitness status. Bodies lacking in energy and racked by pain are themselves stressors, and they significantly interfere with efforts to cope with other stressors. Wellness, on the other hand, prevents the body's condition from becoming another stressor and adds considerably to our general resistance to the hurtful effects of stress. Our lifestyles may contribute to our well-being and life span or may prematurely age us. Exhibit 3–1 offers a global assessment of the effects of lifestyle, heredity, and environmental factors on longevity. Smoking, obesity, sedentariness, alcohol abuse, and emotional dispositions shorten our lives. There is much we can do to add years to our lives and life to our years. The following are suggestions for reaching such higher levels of wellness.

## Stop Chemical Warfare Against the Body.

Certain chemicals used widely by the general public have the ability to trigger the stress response. Nicotine and caffeine both are sympathomimetic drugs, that is they activate the sympathetic nervous system. The sympathetic nervous system is the chief system for bringing on the stress response. Cigarette smoking has been cited by the U. S. Department of Health and Human Services as "the single most avoidable cause of death in the United States." Government figures show that nearly 1,100 people a day, or 400,000 people a year, die from diseases directly related to smoking—and this does not count the damage from secondhand smoke or from smoking during pregnancy.

These chemicals also cause the adrenal glands to produce glucocorticoids, which in turn cause the liver to turn glycogen into glucose (blood sugar). Rapid increases in blood sugar may trigger an overproduction of insulin and, thereby, create hypoglycemia. Hypoglycemia is accompanied by the symptoms of the stress response. A single cigarette increases the production of glucocorticoids by 77 percent. To put this in proper perspective, an acute psychotic attack only increases the glucocorticoid level by 75 percent. It is ironic that smokers often give as their reason for smoking its ability to relax them and help them think better. There is partial truth in this claim since rising blood sugar increases one's sense of well-being and aids concentration. However, rapid increases in blood sugar may create hypoglycemia on the rebound and bring on a nervous condition that is likely to trigger further smoking. In effect, the smoker

(*Text continued on page* 66)

**Exhibit 3-1.** How to Calculate Your Life Expectancy

---

*Instructions.* If you are between 20 and 65 and are reasonably healthy, this test provides a life insurance company's view of your likely longevity.

1. *Start with 72.*
2. *Gender:*
   a. If you are a male, subtract 3.
   b. If you are a female, add 4. (That's right, there is a seven-year spread between the sexes).
3. *Lifestyle:*
   a. If you live in an urban area with a population over two million, subtract 2. If you live in a town under 10,000, or on a farm, add 2. (City life means population, tension).
   b. If you work behind a desk, subtract 3.
   c. If you exercise strenuously (tennis, running, swimming, etc.) five times a week for at least a half hour, add 4. Two or three times a week, add 2.
   d. If you live with a spouse or a friend, add 5. If not, subtract 1 for every ten years alone since age twenty-five. (People together eat better, take care of each other, become less depressed).
4. *Psyche:*
   a. Sleep more than ten hours each night? Subtract 4. (Excessive sleep is a sign of depression, circulatory diseases).
   b. Are you intense, aggressive, easily angered? Subtract 3.
      Are you easygoing, relaxed, a follower? Add 3.
   c. Are you happy? Add 1.
      Are you unhappy? Subtract 2.
   d. Have you had a speeding ticket in the last year? Subtract 1. (Accidents are the fourth-largest cause of death; first, in young adults.)
5. *Success:*
   a. Earn over $50,000.00 a year? Subtract 2. (Wealth breeds high living, tension.)
   b. If you finished college, add 1. If you have a graduate or professional degree, add 2 more. (Education seems to lead to moderation; at least that's the theory).
   c. If you are 65 or over and still working, add 3. (Retirement kills.)
6. *Heredity:*
   a. If any grandparent lived to 85, add 2. If all four grandparents lived to 80, add 6.
   b. If either parent died of a stroke or heart attack before the age of 50, subtract 4
   c. If any parent, brother, or sister under 50 has (or had) cancer or a heart condition, or has had diabetes since childhood, subtract 3.
7. *Health:*
   a. Smoke more than two packs a day? Subtract 8. One to two packs? Subtract 6. One-half to one? Subtract 3.
   b. Drink the equivalent of a qt. of a pint of liquor a day? Subtract 1.

*(Continued on next page)*

**Exhibit 3-1.** (Continued)

---

    c. Overweight by 50 lbs.or more? Subtract 8. Thirty to fifty lbs.?
       Subtract 4. Ten to thirty lbs.or more? Subtract 2.
    d. Men over 40, if you have annual checkups, add 2. Women, if you see
       a gynecologist once a year, add 2.

8. *Age Adjustment:*
    a. Between 30—40? Add 2.
    b. Between 40—50? Add 3.
    c. Between 50—70? Add 4.
    d. Over 70? Add 5.

It's no fun playing the game unless you know how well you've done. The table below tells what percentage of the population, born the same year you were, you will outlive, provided you make it to the specified age. Look across the row of ages and spot the age closest to the age you are "scheduled" to die. Now look down the column. The first figure is the percentage of males whom you will outlive and the second is the percentage of females you will outlive.

| | | | | | AGE | | | | |
|---|---|---|---|---|---|---|---|---|---|
| | 60 | 65 | 70 | 75 | 80 | 85 | 90 | 95 | 100 |
| MALES | 26% | 36% | 48% | 61% | 75% | 87% | 96% | 99% | 100% |
| FEMALES | 15% | 20% | 30% | 39% | 53% | 70% | 88% | 97% | 99.6% |

*Source:* P. Passell. Article appearing in The San Francisco Chronicle and reprinted in B. Combs, D. Hales, and B. Williams, *An Invitation to Health* (Menlo Park, California: Benjamin/Cummings Publishing, 1980), 419–420.

---

*(Text continued from page 64)*
is seeking his or her sugar fix. Caffeine works in the same way, but its effects are considerably weaker. Thus smoking or the heavy use of caffeine will trigger the stress response.

    Aspects of our diet may be stress-inducing. Heavy use of simple sugars, and, to a lesser degree, processed flour may diminish the stock of vitamin C and the B complex vitamins, all crucial to the production of the stress hormones. Nicotine is particularly bad in lowering the body's store of vitamin C. This suggests the possible need for additional amounts of C and B complex vitamins for smokers and sugar addicts. Moreover, heavy use of simple sugars may trigger the stress response in the same way nicotine and caffeine do. Large amounts of simple sugar will create an excessive amount of blood sugar and may bring on hypoglycemia as a rebound effect. The symptoms of hypoglycemia are identical to symptoms of the stress response.

Some persons skip breakfast except for a couple cups of coffee and a cigarette, and by their mid-morning break their blood sugar dips noticeably. To cope with their disturbing weakness they wolf down a sweet roll or two along with more coffee and cigarettes. The result is explosive. They are creating a roller-coaster effect with their blood sugar.

Overall, nutrition may be one of the most neglected inhibitors of disabling stress. The general principles of good nutrition may be easily violated under pressure. Some respond by losing their appetite, others eat too much or incorrectly. Staying in tune with the body is especially important at such times. The old rule of eating a healthy breakfast rich in carbohydrates, protein, and fiber is especially important. Fruits and vegetables are high in essential vitamins and minerals and in fiber, which is necessary for a healthy digestive tract. Moreover, fruits and vegetables are low in fat—an additional plus since high-fat diets have been implicated in heart disease, cancer, and obesity. The best choices seem to be dark green leafy and deep yellow vegetables, potatoes, beans, citrus fruits, melons, and berries. The practice of eating these complex carbohydrates revs up neurotransmitters and hormones that nicely regulate the sympathetic nervous system. If overeating is your reaction to stress, pay close attention to what you eat. Keep a food notebook and favor healthy high-fiber snacks, lots of fruits and vegetables. Drink lots of water—at least eight glasses—each day and avoid beverages containing caffeine or sugar. Focus on a variety of foods and do not skip meals. If stress ruins your appetite, the same rules apply. However, a 50-percent reduction in food for three to five days is harmless. Substituting a commercial liquid shake at one meal can help meet nutrient requirements. With both overeating and appetite loss, moderate exercise such as walking aids digestion, reduces stress, and seems to assist in appetite control.

Excessive drinking of alcohol also may contribute to stress buildup. While its immediate effects may be stress-reducing, its long-range effects may be devastating. The health hazards associated with alcohol abuse will themselves prove stressful. The social fallout of excessive drinking also may prove stressful: for example, loss of a job, family strife, and injury to one's self-esteem.

Some over-the-counter drugs with which many self-medicate also may trigger the stress response. Certain diet pills, for instance, contain amphetamines which are stress-arousing. A number of prescription drugs may trigger the stress response as well. For example, preparations containing thyroxin may prove highly stressful. Recently, one of the authors observed a marked increase in his client's stress symptoms over a three-week period. Nothing in the interview sessions seemed to account for the increased agitation. Because the therapist was aware of the effects of thyroxin and knew the client had been treated in the past for hypothyroidism, he asked if she were presently taking this medication. She said she was and sheepishly confessed that she had significantly increased the dosage without consulting with her internist. She was strongly advised to visit her physician and have her thyroxin level checked. Although agreeing to do so, she delayed her visit for three weeks during which time she returned to her normal dosage. Her agitation steadily decreased during this period. Upon her visit three weeks later, her thyroxin levels were still slightly elevated.

The commonly used sleep potions—barbiturates—can also add indirectly to stress. Barbiturates allow a person to fall asleep quite readily *but they eliminate dreaming from the sleep cycle.* The sleep cycle involves a 60-to-90-minute period of deep sleep during which the brain produces slow waves called *theta* and *delta* followed by a 20-to-30-minute period of dream sleep during which the faster beta and alpha waves are produced. Exhibit 3–2 depicts these waves. The theta-delta deep-sleep periods are associated with physiological recuperation. The deeper the wave the greater the restfulness. Fibromyalgia, a painful condition of the muscle fibers suffered more often by women, has been associated with sleeping patterns with inadequate delta periods. In old age there is a complete absence of delta sleep, and older persons typically complain of a great deal more muscle aches and pains. Antihistamines appear to help the situation somewhat, and aerobic exercise may help markedly.

The 20-to-30-minute periods are dreaming periods accompanied by rapid eye movements (REM) and brain waves made up of alpha and beta. At the beginning of each of these periods there is a penile erection in males and a clitoral engorgement in females. The muscles throughout the body are largely paralyzed during this period. Dreaming sleep appears to be a natural way of de-stressing persons to the previous day's stressful activities. Moreover it appears to be helpful in consolidating short-term memories into long-term ones and in maintaining one's sense of time and space.

Thus it appears that deep sleep is primarily for physiological recuperation, while dreaming appears to have several values for one's emotional and intellectual functions. The barbiturates in sleeping potions eliminate dreaming from the sleep pattern along with its gifts to the psyche. Consequently, persons experiencing stress-induced insomnia should beware of these medications. Because these treatments for insomnia

**Exhibit 3-2.** The Relative Amplitudes and Frequencies of the Four Brain Waves

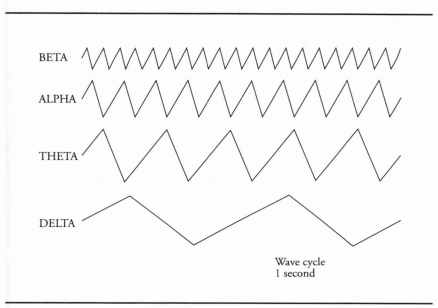

BETA

ALPHA

THETA

DELTA

Wave cycle
1 second

inhibit the dreaming pattern, insomnia is sometimes called the most iatrogenic disease, that is a disease which is worsened by medical treatment.

## Take Up Aerobic Exercise

Walter M. Bortz II, M.D., an expert on aging at Stanford University and the author of *We Live Too Short and Die Too Long* says "Nobody really lives long enough to die of old age. We die from accidents, disease and, most of all, disuse."[1] Most Americans don't burn out, they rust out from inactivity—and recent reports from the President's Council on Fitness suggest that children are in even worse physical shape than their parents. The human body desperately needs activity and exercise; and the exercise that is most vital to our well-being is aerobic exercise.

The word *aerobic* refers to oxygen, and aerobic exercise refers to exercising at a pace wherein the body is taking in roughly as much oxygen as it is using. Upon the completion of the exercise, therefore, there should not be much of an oxygen debt. The formula for computing the heart rate training range is offered in Exhibit 3-3. The figure

**Exhibit 3-3.** Lower and Upper Limits of the Aerobic Training Range

---

220 − Your Age = Max. Heart Rate

Max. Heart Rate × 70% = Lower Limit

Max. Heart Rate × 85% = Upper Limit

---

220 represents the highest heart beat of humans. You must subtract your age from this figure as you lose one maximum heartbeat each year of your life to obtain your present maximum heart rate. You multiply this figure by 60 percent to get the lower limit of your aerobic heart rate training range. To get the upper limit you multiple your present maximum heart rate by 85 percent. Any exercise you engage in (walking, jogging, swimming, stepping, rowing, cycling, aerobic dancing, or whatever) that keeps your heartbeat within this range is considered aerobic. You should continue the exercise for 20 to 30 minutes at least every other day. Aerobic exercise helps prevent serious fallout from stress by increasing energy levels, protecting against heart disease, and decreasing stress hormones.

Virtually all persons can increase their energy levels significantly by beginning an aerobic exercising program. The chief sources of the energy gain are (1) a significant increase in red blood cells that transport oxygen, and (2) an increase in the efficiency of the mitachrondria in using oxygen. The mitachrondria are little factories within cells which mix oxygen with glucose to produce energy. The Academy of Sports Medicine maintains that aerobic exercise will increase the average person's ability to use oxygen by 25 percent. The increase in red blood cells and mitachrondria efficiency improves both our ability to take *in* and to take *up* oxygen.

Aerobic exercise is quite useful in protecting against heart disease. It increases the size and strength of the heart muscle and thus decreases the resting heart rate by improving its per-minute output of blood. This is important because the heart muscle feeds itself blood only between beats. If the heart muscle is weak and inefficient in pumping blood, it must beat so quickly during stress that it will have little time to feed itself. This inability to properly feed itself brings on ischemia, the prelude to a heart attack.

Aerobic exercise significantly changes the concentrations of high- and low-density lipoproteins (HDL and LDL) in a healthy direction. The lipoproteins are fatty protein substances that wrap cholesterol molecules. These molecules attach themselves to arterial lining, forming a kind of sludge that is the beginning of atherosclerosis. The depositing of cholesterol is worsened considerably if the wrapping is done primarily by LDL. The HDL, on the other hand, removes freshly deposited cholesterol molecules from arterial walls. Its action is akin to that of Drain-O™ in cleaning out pipes. Thus, LDL raises the risk of atherosclerosis and HDL decreases it. Aerobic exercise has a pronounced effect on these concentrations. It lowers LDL and raises HDL. Aerobic exercise, then, is the closest thing yet to a magic bullet when it comes to protecting us against heart disease.

Aerobic exercise also rids the body of stress hormones. While the exercise itself produces these hormones, the metabolic fire created by the exercise burns up all the stress hormones it creates plus those previously stored in the body. The reduction in lactic acid is particularly helpful. Lactic acid is known to fatigue muscle tissue and is believed to create a general nervous condition if accumulated in sufficient amounts.

## Avoid Unnecessary Stressors

The lives of some are cluttered with unnecessary tasks that create a sense of overload. This busy lifestyle may serve to make these persons feel important, to ensure them of being productive, or to distract them from issues that are troubling. For whatever reason, this cluttered approach adds considerably to their stress load and should be changed.

### Make Important Life Decisions With Care.

Some life decisions have lasting effects on one's happiness. An unfortunate choice of a spouse, or an occupation, or a major purchase may create an endless string of future stressors. Consequently, the use of proper decision-making skills at such junctures in one's life may prevent much stress later on. Learning these skills and taking the time and energy to use them may yield rich dividends for one's health and happiness.

*"Satisficing" vs. "Optimizing."* Herbert Simon writes of two basic ways of decision making.[2] First, there is "satisficing," that is choosing the first reasonably satisfactory alternative in a problem situation. Second, there is "optimizing," a deliberate, rather exhausting, method of approaching decision making. Simon observes that most persons satisfice most of the time and that this rather sloppy way of making decisions often will do. Indeed, he suggests that it is the preferable mode for most of the

decisions we are called upon to make. However, where the implications of the decision are grave and long-lasting, it is best to optimize.

Optimizing decisions involves carefully defining the problem requiring a decision, establishing criteria for judging alternative solutions, seeking information in order to identify a full array of alternatives, applying the criteria to the alternatives in order to evaluate their merit, selecting an alternative from the array, committing oneself to acting upon the decision, remaining open to feedback regarding the effects of the decision, and recycling to begin the process over again if feedback is sufficiently negative.

*Bases for Inadequate Decisions.* The most common basis for inadequate decision making is the failure to properly define the problem. If we inaccurately define the problem, then *all* alternatives will prove unacceptable. Turn the problem over in your mind and discuss it with trusted friends or professionals to hone in more accurately on the actual dimensions of the problem before trying to solve it.

The second most frequent cause for flawed decisions stems from our failure to *actively* seek alternative solutions. Indecision creates anxiety, and to rid ourselves of the psychic pain we impulsively satisfice the decision. That is, we latch onto the first alternative that has any chance of being satisfactory. Nietzsche said "the first representation that explains the unknown as familiar feels so good that one considers it true."[3] While the immediate result of this impulsivity is often anxiety assuaging, the long-range results may be disastrous.

A third error in problem solving is procrastination in selecting a solution. The procrastination actually may result from a person's unwillingness to give up all other alternatives. A choice *for* one alternative is a choice *against* all other alternatives in one's awareness. The proverbial "cold feet" of the bride on her wedding day may result more from having to give up other suitors than from any concern over the merits of her choice.

The procrastination may also result from fear of having one's choices evaluated by others. Alfred Adler referred to this form of procrastination as *neurotic indecision.* Persons guilty of this kind of indecision often suffer from inferiority complexes that render them hypersensitive to the negative evaluations of others. The unconscious thinking must be "If I don't make decisions, others cannot judge me." This neurotic need to have others approve their every decision will freeze them into inactivity.

## Beware of Empty Ego Struggles

Most human embroilments are empty ego struggles where the only prize is the protection of one's image. We argue about issues that do not *really* matter. The point of the argument is actually to decide who is to be declared the victor, to be declared "right." At such times we act as though we would rather be right than happy. We want to feel a certain way about ourselves, and we insist that others help us by warranting the brittle images we hold for ourselves. If we are constantly caught up in these ego struggles, our self-images are likely to be out of sync with reality.

To prevent stress from these damaging ego struggles, we must establish a more accurate self-image and become comfortable with it. We must put ourselves in proper perspective. Undoubtedly many of us take ourselves too seriously. One disc jockey had it right when he said, "The thing that most determines how many people will attend your funeral is *the weather.*"

## Reduce Noise in Your Life

When noise exceeds 85 decibels, the stress response usually develops.[4] The sound of a motor truck passing is roughly 80 decibels, and the sound of a power mower is approximately 110 decibels. Modern life is extremely noisy both inside and outside of our homes. It appears we are all so junked up on noise that we are uncomfortable with quietude. The thoughtful, serene life will require a certain amount of quietude. We would do well to conduct an audit of our homes to check out the noise levels and make an effort to reduce unnecessary noise.

# Alter Type A Behavior Patterns

In chapter 2, Type A persons were identified as being particularly vulnerable to stress and heart attacks. The lethal formula appears to be busyness combined with cynical distrust, hostility, and anger-in as a means of dealing with one's hostility. The heart of this personality was said to be time urgency. Type A persons were said to suffer from "hurry sickness," to frequently operate under unrealistic time constraints imposed by *themselves.* Because they believe their value derives solely from their productions, they are driven to produce. They feel vaguely anxious when they are not producing. To drown out concerns about their intrinsic worth, they submerge themselves in a myriad of activities, often failing to discriminate between the important and the trivial. This approach to tasks will create a great deal of frustration, and frustration leads to hostility. Consequently, modifying this sense of time urgency should lower one's hostility and thereby reduce one's vulnerability to coronary artery disease.

While these behaviors seem to spring from certain dynamics that do not yield easily to change, concerted efforts to modify them seem in order. If you believe yourself to be a Type A, the following suggestions may be helpful.

## Be Honest With Yourself.

Do you believe your sense of personal worth derives solely from your productions? If you are not producing, do you feel vaguely uncomfortable? Have you unconsciously concluded that you are not natively of value? If you have answered these questions "yes," you are likely to continue feeling pressure to produce virtually every hour of your waking day. This relentless drive to prove your worth by your productions is enormously stressful.

Your drivenness may be so all-encompassing that it robs you of opportunities to become a more complete person. You may be emphasizing *doing* to the exclusion of *being*. One way to feel intrinsically more valuable is to spend more time becoming—becoming an interesting conversationalist, becoming a person with finely honed cultural tastes, becoming an informed person, becoming a person of depth.

## Strengthen the Spiritual Dimensions of Your Life

The word *spiritual* is used to mean many different things. The term is frequently used to refer to a rich interior life—to interests that transcend the busyness of our lives. In this sense it clearly involves clarifying one's values and attempting to bring the movement of one's life on line with them. Excessive busyness interferes with the development of the spiritual dimensions—indeed, it may be a vehicle for keeping us from having to do the hard work necessary for spiritual growth. Busyness to escape the hard work of clarifying our values and of properly ordering our lives brings about a kind of tranquilization of the trivia.

Set aside time daily to sort out your personal values. What is it that you want to do with your life? One way of answering this question is to try to imagine yourself lying on a hospital bed reviewing your past life just hours away from death. How would you have to live your life now in order to feel a sense of integrity in that hour? Clearly identify a few things that would appear to be of paramount importance to you in that hour, and start doing them *now*! Blow away the chaff and make more room in your life for the truly important things.

Humans are doers and problem solvers. The mind is a problem-solving biocomputer—problem solving is what it does best. It is addicted to solving problems, and if it is not presented with problems from the environment, it creates its own so that it can practice solving them. Without disciplining ourselves, we are constantly worrying about things—big things, little things, it doesn't matter. Worry fills the mind like gas fills a container. Just as gas molecules spread out to fill the space whether large or small, worries—however big or little—fill the space in our minds as well. Most of us are Type A in the sense that we are constantly worrying and constantly doing.

When overwhelmed by a spate of tasks, inspect each and ask yourself "In what way is this task contributing to my welfare or the welfare of others?" If you cannot give yourself a satisfactory answer, drop the task from your list. Stop doing things merely because they are there. Remember, nothing is so *inefficient* as doing *efficiently* something that did not need being done in the first place.

Moral philosophy and religious faiths give major attention to values. One field of philosophy, *axiology*, is devoted to the study of values. Another, *epistemology*, is concerned with ways of *knowing*. The two are related inasmuch as our values will reflect the modes of discovering "truth" that we adopt. Hunter Lewis has written a highly readable, most helpful treatise combining axiology and epistemology, titled *A Question of Values*.[5] He surveys the six ways individuals make the personal choices that shape their lives. Each of these ways (dependence on authority, logic, sense experience, emotion, intuition, and science) have their merits. The matrix of factors available to us in sorting out our values is truly complex, and we authors do not have the audacity to prescribe for others what their values should be. However one does it, clarifying one's values is a cardinal requirement for successful decision making.

Once you know what is important to you, insist on spending as much of your time as possible at activities that support these values. If your work seems to have integrity, to have meaning for you, it will be easier for you to commit yourself to it. Susan Kobassa found that commitment to one's work was one of the most effective buffers against stress-induced illness.[6] Work that fits your values will provide you with rich psychological rewards. In searching for such work heed the words of Don Juan when he advised:

> Look at every path closely and deliberately. Try it as many times as you think necessary . . . [Ask yourself], "Does this path have a heart?" If it does, the path is good; if it doesn't, it is of no use. [A path with a heart] makes for a joyful journey . . . [But following a path without a heart] will make you curse your life.[7]

The fullest life cannot be lived without some effort to clarify one's values, to make sense out of the crazy quilt of human experience. Making sense out of things is a human imperative. Kurt Vonnegut made this point when he wrote:

> Tiger got to hunt,
> Bird got to fly;
> Man got to sit and wonder,
>     Why, why, why?
> Tiger got to sleep,
> Bird got to land;
> Man got to tell himself
>     He understand."[8]

## Practice Being Creative When Forced to Wait

Waiting in line or waiting at the doctor's office or being caught up in slow traffic is infuriating to some. Good planning and good assertive skills may help in some cases; nevertheless, there will be many times in which your only realistic alternative will be to wait. You can use these times creatively. Carry interesting reading material with you when visiting your doctor's office. Save some of your favorite musical cassettes for the slow traffic on the freeway. Use the time to plan the rest of your day or to train yourself to get in touch with your body by attending to your sensations. Then congratulate yourself for such a sane approach to an otherwise maddening situation.

## Accept the Fact That Life is Unfinished

The need to hurry up and finish things is highly stressful. At the beginning of *The Tao,* Lau Tsu makes reference to the "ten thousand things." The point is that we tend to get caught up with these ten thousand things and to lose ourselves in the effort to finish them. There always will be ten thousand things, for once we resolve one problem another pops up to take its place. If we worked unrelentingly and finished 9,999 things, we merely would turn around only to find 10,000 more. If we are to experience a sense of self-possession, a sense of inner composure, we must become comfortable with incompleteness. No matter how hard we try, we are going to leave quite a mess of unfinished business when we go. If we wait until the *immediate* is taken care of before beginning the journey to sort out our values, we will never leave the starting gate.

Imagine how ridiculous it would be for a pianist to finish a beautiful concerto as soon as possible! Yet some of us act as though the goal of life is to finish. We should remember that life is a journey, not a destination.

This hurrying approach to our work is worse yet if you add the perfectionist's touch — now it becomes not only to hurry up and finish things but get them *right* as well! Such attitudes add unnecessary grimness to life. To help us counter this pinched-up approach to life someone has written "This life is only a test. If it were a *real* life, we would have been given more information and directions on how to proceed."

Unless we face down this neurotic need to hurry up and finish things, the mindless busyness of our lives will crescendo dangerously, the ten thousand things will consume us. This drivenness to hurry creates an impatience and stressful approach to life. To those suffering from hurry sickness Barry Stevens' book *Don't Push the River* becomes an apt admonition.[9] Those driven to "get it right" should heed Hugh Prather when he said that his life had become happier when he realized that things were *never* quite the way he would like them to be.[10]

The self-defeating approach of persons who are so intent on accomplishing goals that they ignore stress signals is accurately depicted by Paul Newman in the movie, *The Hustler.* As the young pool shark, he was obsessed with the goal of dethroning the king of billiards, Minnesota Fats (Jackie Gleason). In one scene he is competing for high stakes with Minnesota Fats. As the contest wears on throughout the night Newman becomes more and more intense. In his impatience he refuses to eat and his appearance became increasingly unshaven and grim. Minnesota Fats, however, was the consummate professional. He periodically retreated to the wash room to shave and groom himself. Newman's unrested machine eventually broke down under the strain, while Minnesota Fats ended the game with enviable aplomb.

## Don't Fight the Clock

Type A persons think the hands on the clock move more slowly than they do. They incessantly overcommit themselves, and their self-imposed time limits are impossible to meet. They grossly underestimate the amount of time it takes to complete tasks. These unrealistic time estimates leave them angered by their "slowness." More realistic planning would save them from a great deal of stress. They need to develop more respect for the complexity of tasks they take on and much more tolerance for unanticipated hurdles that arise. One way to handle impatience is to allow an indefinite time for each job (or at least double the amount of time estimated for its completion).

Impatience is often a sign that one is not invested in the activity. Because Type A's are addicted to getting things done, they may exercise little choice over *what* they do. Consequently, they often may find themselves frantically working at things that are of little consequence to them. Their basic goal at such times is merely to finish, to move on to other things. With little investment in the task, every unexpected interference is experienced as a major barrier put in the way by some malevolent fiend. The antidote for this impatience is to make more conscious choices of tasks, to eliminate trivial busywork, and to save time and energy for tasks that really matter. Learning to say "No" is of great help in clearing out tasks that are not personally rewarding.

One of the authors who is a bonafide, card-carrying member of the Type A species had an experience a few years past that depicts his problem with fighting the clock. One afternoon he set out to wallpaper his son's bedroom. His wife asked him when he wanted to eat supper. Noticing it was 3:15 in the afternoon, he said "What about 6:30?" She said "OK," and then added parenthetically, "Now you know you won't be through by 6:30." Feigning ignorance of her meaning, he replied "Why?" "Because you won't, that's why. You can't wallpaper a room in three hours and fifteen minutes," she said somewhat exasperated. Accepting the challenge he said, "Oh, yeah. You have supper ready and you'll see." But 6:30 came and went and the hours wore on until at 1:00 a.m. he put up the last strip of paper a bit diagonally. But by that time he did not care, for he was so angry with his "incompetence" that he could have eaten nails — and he should have because he hadn't yet eaten his supper!

This story demonstrates the height of neuroticism. Here was a man doing a job under self-imposed time constraints, feeling behind and out of sorts all the while. The really disturbing thing is that nobody on the planet even cared when he finished. Moreover, his son didn't even want his room wallpapered in the first place. He didn't want his wall stickers covered up. So the man is doing it for himself, on his own time schedule, and feeling angry and hopelessly behind schedule all the while. (Incidentally, the author promises the reader that he has made some progress in changing this behavior; however, discount his wife's opinion were you to speak with her about this matter).

## Pace Your Efforts

Pace your efforts so you do not work in spasms. Paul Simon said it nicely in the song "Feeling Groovy": "Slow down, you move too fast. You've got to make the morning last." The goal is not to shirk your duties but rather to do them with some degree of centeredness, to remain reasonably calm and collected while focusing on one task at a time.

## Renegotiate Deadlines With Others

Persons suffering from hurry sickness are reluctant to ask that deadlines be extended. They view such requests as evidence of their incompetence, disorganization, or sloth. Consequently, they frantically push ahead trying desperately to finish on time. To protect their egos, they are willing to put their bodies under great strain. In reality, renegotiation is a legitimate and acceptable way of handling multiple responsibilities. It is often expected and acceptable to others. Learning to renegotiate, then, is an effective tool for lowering stress.

# Eliminate Anxious Reactive Behaviors

As mentioned in chapter 2, anxious reactive persons magnify the effect of stressors in two ways. First, they get nervous over getting nervous; that is, their awareness of stress symptoms becomes yet another stressor. Second, they mentally rehearse stressful situations over and over. The first step in changing this adjustment is to become conscious of the behavior. Realize that you are heaping stress upon stress. Catch yourself in the act and use your awareness of stress symptoms to cue more functional behaviors such as regulated breathing and on-task focusing. Donald Meichenbaum's Stress Inoculation technique offers a step-by-step approach for handling stressors in this functional manner.[11]

# Deconditioning Hypersensitivities

The stress response is sometimes automatically triggered by conditioned stimuli such as phobias. Fear of heights, fear of closed or open spaces, fear of authority figures, fear of flying, fear of examinations, and fear of public speaking may all reach phobic levels. A kind of radical surgery is necessary wherein the person must be deconditioned to these stimuli. The most common form of deconditioning is systematic desensitization, a procedure whereby images of the feared experience are associated with feelings of deep relaxation. In this way these images lose their ability to elicit the unpleasant emotional sensations. While there are automated, self-administered forms of systematic desensitization, it is generally best to seek professional assistance for these problems.[12] The procedure is quite effective and usually takes anywhere from ten to fifteen sessions.

# Develop a Sense of Control

The previous chapter emphasized the critical importance of a sense of control over one's life. Both animal and human studies strongly suggest that it is the *un*controllable event that does the damage. In one study, the correlation between events perceived to be within the control of the person and subsequent illness was actually *zero!*[13] On the other hand, the correlation between events beyond one's control and illness was highly significant. It is the perception of control, and not necessarily the reality of control, that makes the difference. Consequently, increasing a sense of control will lower one's vulnerability to stress-induced illness.

## Acknowledge the Control You Do Have

One way of increasing a sense of control is to become aware of the extent to which *we* are initiating events in our lives. We tend to blame others for life's pressures, yet informal surveys suggest that upwards of 75 percent of life events are self-initiated. Thus, "they" are not doing it to us; *we* are doing it to us! Realizing this will help us to feel more in control of events, even if we do not enjoy them.

## Use Your Control in Making Choices

One way of empowering oneself is to insist on making choices for oneself. Choice-making is a god-like quality within us. The difference between human androids and human beings is the human being's ability to make choices based on a shifting background of values. With the advancement of artificial intelligence, androids can be programmed to take a larger matrix of factors into consideration, but the difference between them and us is still astronomical. Choosing is our crowning ability, and making choices is self-empowering.

## Maintain Stimulation Within Your Optimal Range

We sense things are out of control when the demand load becomes excessive. There appears to be for each of us a range of stimulation that is optimal. The optimal stimulation range is that range of stimulation within which we function best. Optimal does not mean maximal nor minimal; it means the most *favorable* level of stimulation. It is one's comfort zone in handling demands. When stimulation falls comfortably within this range, we tend to flow with our work, our mood states are upbeat, and we experience a general sense of well-being. Stimulation exceeding the range triggers the symptoms of overchallenge, while those undershooting the range trigger boredom. Exhibit 3–4 depicts the relationship between demand levels and coping.

The test for determining one's optimal stimulation range is personal and subjective. Perhaps the reader has some general idea of that point in demand buildup where one begins to show stress symptoms—where one experiences unsteady attention, an intolerance for any interruptions, and a general sense of malaise. At the other end of the demand continuum you may be aware of those times when too little is going on, when you need more rather than less to perk you up. Obviously these measurements are inexact; but some careful attention to body sensations when experiencing various levels of stimulation can sharpen one's awareness of the optimal range.

Unfortunately, most persons pay little attention to body sensations. They ignore such signals in the interest of pushing ahead with their ego pursuits. Consequently, they miss vital information from their best friend—their body—regarding the proper match between demands and coping resources. If you believe you ignore these vital signs, begin the practice of body scanning. We commonly ask others how they feel but fail to ask ourselves. Form the habit of frequently scanning body sensations for clues as to the appropriateness of the demand load. What is your body telling you at this moment? Have you been reading too long without a break? Are your eyes tired? Your upper shoulders and neck

**Exhibit 3-4.** The Relationship Between Demand Level and Coping

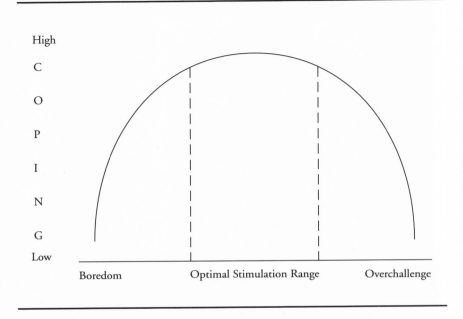

tense from holding this book too long? Forming the habit of body scanning is not easy; it will take considerable time and effort.

As we pointed out in the previous section, we have much more control than we sometimes believe. It is easier to fault the elusive "they" than to take responsibility for excessive demands. Quite simply, if demands seem especially burdensome, look for opportunities to delegate some and drop others. Take action to ensure that the demand load falls comfortably within your optimal range. If you are experiencing serious stressors at work, save the divorce until next year!

In one sense, many of us do not make many choices. That is, we are so well programmed by our enculturation that we fly on automatic pilot most of the time. Much of our behavior is reflexive and prescribed. We have given over the controls too completely to the automatic pilot. A kind of repetition compulsion takes over, making life seem unreal—like a rerun. While automating responses frees up our consciousness for other functions, living too reflexively gives a dream-like quality to our lives. Taking the controls and consciously making decisions causes us to feel powerful. The resulting sense of control over our lives is an effective buffer against crippling stress symptoms.

# Increase Coping Resources

Increasing one's coping resources will positively impact the demands-resources equation and eliminate considerable stress. A useful step in improving resources is first to diagnose them. *The Coping Resources Inventory for Stress (CRIS)* is a highly useful inventory for this purpose.[14] It measures fifteen coping resources, identifies strengths and weaknesses, and offers recommendations for improving deficits. With such information one can direct efforts at self-change more precisely.

## Credit Yourself for Resources You Already Have

Another way of increasing a sense of control is to honestly credit yourself for those coping resources that you *already* possess. Many people underestimate their resources. When challenged, they begin a series of negative self-statements such as, "I've never been good at this. Why do I let myself in for this sort of thing?" or "I can't handle this! What am I going to say to others when they discover I've failed?" Such pejorative self-talk steals their energy, diverts their attention from critical aspects of the situation, and stresses them out. If such "poor mouthing" has become habitual, it will require concerted effort to effectively counter it. If you are afflicted with such self-defeating mental habits, you would do well to commit yourself to the serious work of reprogramming your self-image.

## Strengthening the Self-Image

Acceptance, confidence, and self-directedness are powerful resources for coping with stress. Their effects on coping are perhaps more pervasive than any other resource. *Acceptance* is a matter of respecting and liking oneself. Acceptance implies a tolerance of mistakes and foibles in oneself and comes from challenging perfectionistic parts of oneself that are highly critical. *Confidence* is having faith in one's abilities to deal effectively with life. *Self-directedness* reflects the decision to trust one's *own* wisdom in running one's life. Obviously these traits represent rather consistent ways of perceiving oneself. As mentioned in chapter 1, Bem suggests that we get our self concepts from what we *see ourselves doing*.[15] Consequently, if we wish to adopt more positive views of ourselves, we must direct our attention to our more laudable traits. We are not referring to a kind of narcissistic pride that the theologists call *hubris*, but rather to taking pride or pleasure in the creditable aspects of one's behavior. The direction of one's attention is the primary tool for changing one's identity. There are two principle ways to change the views we have of ourselves:

(1) *Passively Notice Negative Self-Talk*. Simply notice each time you are putting yourself down — *without evaluating your self-talk!* Record in a few words the theme of the self-put-down (for example, "am unattractive," "put things off," "didn't speak up for myself.") Merely note the put-down and say to yourself something like, "I seem to want to focus my attention on my shortcomings at the moment. It's all right. I'll just wait until the critical part of me has had its say," Then just listen to yourself. Do *not* get angry with yourself for getting angry with yourself. This only adds fuel to the fire. Est (now called the Forum) says, "Whatever you resist, persists."[16] If you resist your negative self-evaluations, you further energize them. The best approach is merely to notice them. Assume the role of a dispassionate observer and merely watch such negative thoughts cross the stage of your mind.

It's a paradox, but quite often the best way to stop self-critical thoughts is to give yourself over to them — *but be aware of doing so!* Est also cryptically says, "Experiencing experience disappears it."[17] Most of us have had the experience of having a few bars of music obsessively monopolize our attention. Efforts to drive out the music often fail. In such cases it is best to give yourself over to the music — just say to yourself "For some reason I seem to want to sing the song," and do so. Shortly you will become bored with the repetitious strain and it will drop out of your consciousness. Fritz Perls says the way to get rid of unfinished business is to deal with it — stay with the thought — don't try to resist it.[18] That is all! Continue this passive approach to thought control for two weeks or more, and you are likely to discover that critical thoughts occupy less and less of your time. For best results, combine the passive approach with the following active one.

(2) *Actively Reprogram Your Self-Image*. Establish the practice of reviewing your positive resources during periods of relaxation. Relaxation is useful in preparing your mind for self-reprogramming. Virtually every effort at brainwashing begins with a trance-like state, an altered state of consciousness, which can be induced through relaxation as well as other means. One's sense of identity depends largely on the constancy of the stimulation one experiences. Consequently, greatly increasing or

decreasing stimulation lessens the rigidity of one's identity and renders the person more reprogrammable.

*First*, construct a menu of your personal characteristics that please you when you are feeling good, for you are likely to be more generous (and honest) at this time. If you have formed the habit of being highly self-critical, this will not be an easy task. Examine your behaviors, your attitudes toward life, your modes of interacting with others, your job-related, school-related, or family-related roles for evidences of positive characteristics and behaviors. Briefly write down these characteristics.

*Second,* alter your consciousness through a relaxation procedure such as Deep Muscle Relaxation, the Quietening Response, Autogenic Training, or the Relaxation Response, all discussed in the next chapter. Deep states of relaxation alter your consciousness in such a way that your sense of identity is less resistive to change. (It is more difficult to assume new views of oneself in one's normal state of consciousness.) Once in a softened mental state, review your resources in specific detail. It is not enough to think abstractly about personal assets. You must visualize them in detail, see yourself in real-life situations using the assets.

*Third,* after 20 to 30 minutes of serene relaxation, focus your attention of your list of esteemed characteristics. It is very important that you visualize yourself demonstrating these characteristics. It is not useful to think of these characteristics in the abstract. For instance, if you wish to see yourself as a more confident person, you should see yourself behaving confidently. You may be able to think of actual situations in which you have shown great confidence. It may be that you *are* confident in certain spheres of your life but are apprehensive in others. First, visualize repeated instances of your confident behavior, then go on to imagine yourself performing confidently in situations in which you are normally insecure. It is critical that you fill out your picture with great detail. Vagueness will weaken the effect. If imagining yourself giving a speech, look out over your imaginary audience, see the conference room, notice the podium on which your notes rest, and so forth.

These two procedures—objectively noticing your negative self-references and actively attempting to reprogram yourself—will prove helpful in replacing self-defeating ways of thinking. Try out these procedures for a few weeks and experience the satisfaction of rebirthing yourself in a more honest, self-facilitative way. Do not expect overnight miracles in using these techniques. It took many years to forge your present self-image, and change comes slowly—even with good maps and good strategies. Still, few feelings are more rewarding than the sense of personal power that comes from taking oneself in tow and successfully changing self-defeating attitudes and behaviors.

## Learn Tension-releasing Procedures

Stress monitoring, tension control, and cognitive restructuring are coping resources useful in lowering stressful arousal. Tension control, the ability to lower unnecessary arousal, and cognitive restructuring, the ability to control thinking to maintain one's composure, can be improved by practicing the relaxation procedures and mind control suggestions offered in chapter 4.

*Stress Monitoring.* Stress monitoring skills serve a reconnaissance function. They help you to recognize (a) signs of early stress buildup, (b) situations in which you normally feel resourceless, and (c) persons in whose presence you stress yourself out. To improve these skills, practice body scanning. The body is an accurate barometer of stress buildup. It is continually sending a rich set of biofeedback to inform us of how we are responding to our current situations. We typically try to ignore body signals in the interest of our ego pursuits. In stridently marching toward these ego goals, we often drag our bodies over beds of hot coals. The body for the longest while is overly respectful in sending signals. It merely whispers with the help of a headache, backache, or pounding heart. If we fail to take corrective action to remedy our stressful adjustment, the chronic arousal eventually will bring on psychophysiological disorders of more serious magnitude. We must change our attitude toward the body. We must no longer view our efforts to ignore arousal as evidence of self-control, but rather of dysfunctionality. We must see the body as a friend intent on insuring that we properly understand what is happening to us. We go throughout the day asking others how they are without once asking ourselves how *we* are. Body scanning requires focusing attention of the various parts of the body for signs of tension.

*Tension Control and Cognitive Restructuring.* Tension control procedures include prescribed breathing, deep muscle relaxation, and the relaxation response. Cognitive restructuring is an effort to change the meaning that events have for us in order to lower painful arousal. Thus, cognitive restructuring is an approach to mind control.

## Social Support

One can spread the shock of stressful events by obtaining social support through a network of caring others. The creation of such a network depends in part on practicing friendship skills. Primary among these skills is active listening, a serious effort to hear what others are saying and to assure them of your understanding.

# Achieving Serene State of Consciousness

Many persons suffer chronically from stressful mind-sets. They are often dissatisfied with their conditioned way of viewing things and with their negative emotional moods. They are bullied by their feverish, pushy mental states and suffer from a scatterbrainedness that diffuses their attention and dilutes their efforts. They feel like sensory-bound rats, or hyperactive children, who reflexively attend to *whatever* stimulates their senses. Their attention is directed first here and then there. It is as though the mind is running the show independently of the will. They long for more inner peace, more freedom from their conditioning.

This scatterbrainedness is similar to electrical short-circuiting — crazy, high-intensity energy that gets nothing done. St. Teresa in the Middle Ages referred to this *un*disciplined mind as an "unbroken horse." This mental state leaves persons feeling little control over their minds. They intuitively know that there is a more centered, composed state of mind to be experienced but feel cut off from it. They know it is there but cannot bring it into clearly into focus.

Religions throughout history have been concerned with the fragmented nature of human experience and have prescribed ways of reconnecting, of becoming whole again. Indeed, the word *religion* etymologically means "to connect again or to bind back." The word *god* is used for that "something" that is significant to we humans. Religions, then, are primarily concerned with the human being's relationship to this something that is felt to be truly significant. They attempt to help us to experience union with the significant, and thereby, to rid ourselves of estrangement, isolation, and loneliness.

Many religious practices seem designed to bring about an altered state of consciousness; to help us to change our view of nature and our place in it. This altered state is referred to in the East as *enlightenment, samadhi,* or *satori.* In Christian literature it is referred to as "being born again." It is an innocency of perception, a perception stripped of conditioned artificiality. In the New Testament it is said to be a reward unattainable "except ye become as a small child." Again in the New Testament we are admonished "Be not conformed to the world, but be ye transformed by the renewing of your minds." This state is attained only by those who rise above the constraining elements of their enculturation.

In studying what it means to be supranormal, both Abraham Maslow and Jiddu Krisnamurti associate such a state with rebelling against the narrowness of the vision dictated by cultural indoctrination.[19] Mystics often report that things look different, that the boundary between the observer and the object appears to blur, and that they feel a sense of oneness with the objects they are experiencing.

We are often tyrannized by our needs. These tyrants exhaust our energy and monopolize our attention. They cause us to look out at the world with selective perception—we see only those things that have relevance for these needs. In the East such a mental state is referred to as *little mind*. We get all caught up with our egotistical goals, shut up inside our little minds, and miss much of what is beautiful and ennobling in the world. Our entrapment is worsened by our constant talking—talking to others or talking to ourselves. It is difficult to listen when we are talking. Consequently, if we want to tune in to what is happening, we must stop the incessant talking and still the mind with healing silence.

## Thinking Versus Awareness

Zen literature points up a basic incompatibility between thinking (talking to ourselves) and awareness. Developmentally, awareness is primary, while thinking is secondary. In thinking, we use categories. The use of categories becomes a mental shorthand, allowing us to process large quantities of observations economically. This shorthand is efficient; it allows us to communicate quickly with ourselves and with others about a wide range of topics. But we engage in gross "rounding off" errors when we force objects and events into ready-made categories.

As we grow older, more and more is demanded of us, and the use of these abstract categories becomes more and more important. Consequently, the original order of awareness and thinking becomes reversed: thinking now becomes primary, and awareness is reduced to a secondary function. We are aware of an object only long enough to see it as an instance of some category we have in mind. All the uniqueness of the object is lost in the rush to categorize and use it.

In a sense we become prisoners of our mental conditioning, of our need to neatly categorize things; we become less open to new experiences. We are in touch with our environment only through preconceived, and sometimes erroneous, impressions of it. Experiences become so routine, so automatic, that we seldom feel vibrantly alive.

Past conditioning results in standard ways of viewing experience. The rapid and often careless assignment of potentially new experiences to ready-made categories shuts us off to these new experiences. As a result, there is a predictable sameness to experiencing. More and more experiences take on the quality of playbacks or reruns. The novelty and freshness of experience disappears, and we are consigned to live in gray-land. We need to take over from the automatic pilot more often, or as Henry David Thoreau said, to live *deliberately*.[20] This approach requires significant changes in our consciousness.

## Consciousness Raising

The West is currently rediscovering the religio-therapeutic practices of the East. While certain trailblazers such as William James, Ralph Waldo Emerson, Henry David Thoreau, and Carl Jung attempted to translate these practices into Western frames, the richness of Eastern myth and methods has remained relatively obscure to most Westerners.

America was far too busy shaping and bending the external environment to share the concern of the East for the delicate nature of the internal environment. While the West was busy mastering the external world, the East was at work mastering the internal one. This gave them quite a head start toward the new spiritual frontier, the conquest of the inner world.

For most of this century American psychology had largely abandoned the study of consciousness and ignored the exploration of inner space. Out of its insecurity as a science, American psychology identified with the experimental methods of the physical sciences. It was committed to logical positivism, a philosophy of science that asserts that no subject is worthy of investigation that cannot be studied via one of the five senses. If we cannot see it, hear it, feel it, smell it, or taste it, for scientific purposes it does not exist. With the growth of the Human Potential Movement, however—and more recently of transpersonal psychology— this situation is changing. Once again, private experience is becoming a legitimate subject for investigation.

## Meditation

The part of this Eastern practice that is of most interest to us is meditation. Meditation is a vehicle for consciousness-raising. It alters one's consciousness and allows one to transcend the limitations of everyday experiencing. While meditation is practiced in some sects of Christianity and Judaism, it is more widely practiced in Eastern religions. Claudio Naranjo and Robert Ornstein point out that there are many variations in the practice of meditation:

> Thus, while certain techniques (like those in the Tibetan Tantra) emphasize mental images, others discourage paying attention to any imagery; some involve sense organs and use visual forms (mandalas) or music, others emphasize a complete withdrawal from the senses; some call for complete inaction, and others involve action (mantra), gestures (mudra), walking, and other activities. Again, some forms of meditation require the summoning up of specific feeling states, while others encourage an indifference beyond the identification with any particular illusion.[21]

*Hooking the Mind.* To meditate is to dwell upon something. The something is usually a sound (mantra) or a visual figure (mandala). Most people will find it easier to focus upon a sound than on a visual figure. We tend to be visually oriented and, therefore, find it difficult to screen out visual activity. Transcendental meditation followers suggest that it is important to choose the right sound. For this purpose they go back to the Hindu Vedic literature. The words selected tend to be those that set up a vibration that can be felt in the cheek bones, words with the consonants "m," "n," "h," or "ng"; sharp sounds such as "k" or "ch" are avoided. The mantras tend to be euphonious and rhythmical. Examples of common mantras are "om," "aum," "shiam," and "aing." A special feature of such sounds is that they require little effort to make.

In meditation we attempt to drown out distracting thoughts. In repeating the mantra, we soon enough become habituated to it, but we may still be paying enough attention to it for it to fully occupy the mind. Every thought is accompanied by weak muscle activity, that is, the thought causes limited firing of neurons which terminate in muscle tissue. The firing may not be enough to cause visible movements, but it does use energy, and it does involve muscle contraction. If we can preempt tension-arousing thoughts by tying up the mind with low intensity data, muscle tension is reduced, and profound relaxation takes over. In chapter 4 a step-by-step procedure for experiencing one form of meditation, the Relaxation Response, is presented.

*Meditation, a Kind of Neural Inhibitor.* Meditation has an effect upon the body similar to that of a neural inhibitor. In order for a neuron to fire, to send its electrical charge across the gap between itself and the other neurons, it must have the services of a neural transmitter—a chemical that bridges the gap. The hormonal and neurological changes accompanying stress appear to increase the supply of these neural transmitters. The result is a wild twitching of the neurons. A neural inhibitor neutralizes the effects of transmitters and terminates the wild firing. Sedatives and tranquilizers are used extensively to inhibit firing, but some are addictive and many have side effects. Meditation, however, appears to slow down the wild firing in a very natural and healthy way. It involves no outside chemicals, no trauma to the system, no negative side effects, and it results in a healthy addiction (if we are lucky).

*Passive Attitude.* Perhaps the most important ingredient in the formula for inducing the meditative state is a passive attitude. We are to "let go," to "go negative," to "not try." The Zen roshis advise, "Gentle is the way." We are not to fight extraneous thoughts. If our minds wander, we merely return to the silent repetition of the mantra. Very often, beginners complain that they are unable to keep their attention focused on the mantra. They are instructed, however, to stop worrying, to merely be aware of their wandering thoughts, and to gently bring their attention back to the mantra.

*A General Form of Desensitization.* Daniel Goleman refers to meditation as a "natural, global self-desensitization."[22] According to him, we become aware that the mind has wandered when the thoughts and images threaten the state of relaxation. There may be a kind of built-in "relaxostat" that makes us aware of wandering thoughts when they threaten to disturb a state of relaxation. If this is the case, the mind wandering may actually desensitize us to anxious thoughts by associating them with the feeling of deep relaxation and thereby lead to a less stressful life.

An important goal of meditation is the expansion of awareness, liberation from stressful, conditioned thinking. Concentrative forms of meditation seek to focus the mind on the smallest possible target so that awareness can expand. During meditation, awareness precludes thinking. The goal is single-minded attention, a sense of being in touch moment after moment, a sustained openness to the present. The tumultuous waves stirred up by the thinking processes must be calmed, and the mind must become a stilled lake, so it can faithfully mirror its surroundings.

The normal churning condition of the mind militates against serenity. There are too many waves, too much short-circuiting, too much twitching. In this condition the mind is not a friend. Eastern mystics compared it to a drunken monkey, doing all sorts of crazy, useless things. We discover this all too well when we attempt to meditate. We are likely to find it extremely difficult to focus on any target for long. Once the mantra is started, attention flits back and forth over an endless array of nonsense.

If we can stop thinking for awhile, we may be able to expand awareness. Perhaps then we can have a new, more direct experience of reality. The goal of meditation is to stop conditioned thinking and to expand awareness. The Hindu swami, Patanjali, around 150 B.C., wrote: "Yoga is the stopping of the spontaneous activities of the mind." Fritz Perls, the founder of Gestalt therapy, said that the goal of therapy is to "lose your mind to gain your senses."[23]

## Present Centeredness

A lot of stress results from vain imaginings and fretful worrying about future events. Perls defined anxiety as "the gap between the now and the then."[24] The antidote for anxiety is staying in the present. Very few situations are as fearful as our anticipations of them. Consequently, if we can practice taking things one at a time, if we stay with the present moment, we will rid ourselves of a great deal of unnecessary stress.

We have a natural tendency to ignore painful emotions. Yet, suppressing these emotions sometimes prolongs their existence. It is generally better to "stay with the feeling," as the Gestalt therapist is apt to say. When the full heat of attention is directed at the feeling, it will sometimes melt. This is the approach taken by many Filipinos in dealing with the pain of a headache. The sufferer is urged to direct his attention *to* the pain signal and ask himself questions such as the following? "Where is it hurting, exactly where? Does it come and go, or is it constant? What can the pain be compared to?" It sometimes seems that pain signals persist until they are assured that their messages are received and decoded by the executive brain. Suppressing these signals may only prolong them. It is better to recognize them and perhaps even to amplify them temporarily.

Staying with our experiencing in the present moment implies faith in our coping abilities. To dodge present signals or to mentally rehearse future adjustments so completely that the future is shoved into the secure past is a vote of "no confidence" in our resources. We are not suggesting that people abandon themselves to their impulses but rather that they stay in the present and avoid the habit of endlessly processing fearful future events.

Being present means making fresh contact with the now and the ordinary. The good life is to be found in the here and now, not in the there and then. The there and then constitute the Great Illusion made up of fantasized, romantic notions about how life should be. Attention should be directed to the obvious. Awareness of the obvious requires suppression of fantasized future scenarios, reminiscences of the past, and feverish conceptual activity. In truth, the past exists only in our memories, the future only in our plans. The present is our *only* reality! Many poets and writers of sacred literature have written about the importance of living in the present. The poet Longfellow wrote:

> Trust no future, howe'er pleasant,
> Let the dead Past bury its dead!
> Act, act in the living Present! ·
> Heart within and God o'erhead.

In the *Pali Canon* Buddha says, "Do not hark back to things that passed, and for the future cherish no fond hopes." The New Testament quotes Jesus as saying, "Take, therefore, no thought of the morrow, for the morrow shall take thought for the things of itself." And Emerson said:

> These roses under my window make no reference to former roses or to better ones; they are for what they are; they exist with God today. There is not time to them. There is simply the rose; it is perfect in every moment of its existence . . . but man postpones and remembers. He cannot be happy and strong until he, too, lives with nature in the present, above time.

Present-centeredness implies deep involvement in what we are doing at the moment. Robert Pirsig in *Zen and the Art of Motorcycle Maintenance* was to equate this involvement with quality, a characteristic grossly missing in much of what is produced today.[25] The early Greek Sophists referred to involvement when they spoke of "arete." The Shakers believed in the religious value of "concentrated labor," of focusing their attention on their work. The Buddhist tradition suggests that everyday activities should be pursued with "bare attention," attention uncluttered by regrets from the past or worries about the future.

Present-centeredness, detached awareness, involvement in our present actions — these are the altered forms of consciousness pursued by the meditative arts. This unhurried, serene, celebrative attitude toward the present is a splendid antidote for the stressful kind of existence so typical of modern living.

# Summary

Stress is an inevitable condition of life. It is the body's response to any perceived threat, loss, or frustration. Mismanaged stress can seriously injure our health, interfere with smooth personal relationships, lower our work performance, and markedly erode the quality of our lives. There is some evidence to suggest that conditions of high demand may actually *fortify* one's immunological defenses if one feels control over them. There is strong evidence on the other hand that demands perceived as being beyond one's control may lower immunological defenses.

Comprehensive stress management includes both efforts to prevent stressors and to manage them once they have been encountered. Wise living will prevent many stressors. Preventive efforts will include strengthening resistance factors through wellness practices, avoiding unnecessary stressors, altering stress-inducing behavior patterns, building additional coping resources, developing a sense of control, and striving for a more serene state of consciousness.

## ENDNOTES

1. Walter Bortz, *We Live Too Short and Die Too Long: How To Achieve and Enjoy Your Natural 120 Year Lifespan*, (New York: Bantam, 1991).

2. Herbert A. Simon, *The New Science of Management Decision,* rev. ed.(New York: Harper and Row, 1977).

3. F. Nietzsche, "Twilight of the Idols," in *The Portable Nietzsche*, ed. and trans. W. Kaufman (New York: Viking Press, 1954), 497.

4. Jerrold S. Greenberg, *Comprehensive Stress Management* (Dubuque, Iowa: William C. Brown, 1990), 85.

5. Hunter Lewis, *A Question of Values* (New York: Harper Collins, 1990).

6. S. C. Kobassa, "Stressful Life Events, Personality, and Health: An Inquiry into Hardiness," *Journal of Personality and Social Psychology* 37 (1979): 1–11.

7. Carlos Castenada, *A Separate Reality: Further Considerations with Don Juan* (New York: Pocket Books, 1972), 38.

8. Kurt Vonnegut, *Cat's Cradle* (New York: Delta/Seymour Lawrence Book, 1986), 150.

9. Barry Stevens, *Don't Push the River* (Berkeley, California: Celestial Arts, 1985).

10. Hugh Prather, *Notes to Myself* (Moab, Utah: Real People Press, 1970).

11. Donald H. Meichenbaum, "A Self-Instructional Approach to Stress Management: A Proposal for Stress Inoculation Training," in *Stress and Anxiety*, vol. 2, ed. I. Sarason and C. D. Spielberger (New York: Wiley, 1975).

12. S. B. Cotler, "Sex Differences and Generalization of Anxiety Reduction with Automated Desensitization and Minimal Therapist Interaction," *Behaviour Research and Therapy* 8 (1970): 273–285.

13. Kenneth B. Matheny and Penny Cupp, "Control, Desirability, and Anticipation As Moderating Variables between Life Change and Illness," *Journal of Human Stress* 9 (1983): 14–23.

14. Kenneth B. Matheny, William L. Curlette, David W. Aycock, James L. Pugh, and Harry F. Taylor, *The Coping Resources Inventory for Stress* (Atlanta, Georgia: Health PRISMS, Inc., 1987).

15. Daryl Bem, "Self-perception Theory," in *Psychotherapy: Theory Research, and Practice,* vol. 6, ed. L. Berkowitz (New York: Academic Press, 1972).

16. C. Frederick, *Est: Playing the Game the New Way,* (New York: Dell, 1974), 17.

17. Ibid., 26.

18. Fritz Perls, "Four Lectures," in *Gestalt Therapy Now*, ed. Joan Fagan and Irma L. Shepherd (New York: Harper and Row, 1970), 16.

19. Abraham H. Maslow, *The Farther Reaches of Human Nature* (New York: Viking, 1971); Jiddu Krishnamurti, *The Network of Thought* (New York: Harper and Row, 1964).

20. Henry David Thoreau. "Walden," in *The World in Literature,* vol. II, ed. G. K. Anderson and R. Warnock (Glenview, Illinois: Scott, Foresman, 1967), 395.

21. Claudio Naranjo and Robert E. Ornstein, *On the Psychology of Meditation* (New York: Viking Press, 1971), 7.

22. Daniel Goleman, "Meditation Helps Break the Stress Spiral," *Psychology Today* (February 1971): 4–6.

23. Perls, "Four Lectures."

24. Ibid.

25. Robert M. Pirsig, *Zen and the Art of Motorcycle Maintenance* (New York: Bantam Books, 1974).

# CHAPTER FOUR

# TAMING THE STRESS MONSTER

Fight for your highest attainable aim
But never put up resistance in vain.
——Hans Selye, *Stress Without Distress*

If one man conquers in a battle a
thousand times a thousand men,
And if another conquers himself,
he is the greatest of conquerors.
——Buddha

At times our efforts to prevent stress will fail, and we will be caught up in its sticky web. Once the stress is under way, strategies for combating the stressor are in order. These strategies include: (1) obtaining an accurate appraisal of stressors and resources, (2) deciding whether to live with the stressor or try to eliminate it, (3) changing stressful mind-sets, and (4) reducing arousal.

## Accurately Appraising Stressors and Resources

While stress creates hypervigilance, it actually *shrinks* the scope of our attention. We narrowly focus on stressors and attend to them only in the most general way. We are less likely to see the difference between the actual stressor and the exaggerated versions we create in our minds. Rather, we act upon some distorted view of the situation, a view borne more out of our past experiences than from any rigorous inspection of the stressor itself. Successful stress management requires the constructive focusing of one's attention. In the early phases of stress combat,

97

attention should be directed to signs of stress buildup and to an honest appraisal of the stressor and one's resources for coping with it.

## Monitoring Stress Buildup

Recognizing early signs of stress buildup allows us to deal with the situation before the stress escalates to catastrophic proportions. In a study of the effect of self-awareness on illness, Suls and Fletcher found that stressful life events predicted subsequent illness among persons low in private self-consciousness (self-monitoring) but not in persons high in private self-consciousness.[1] Body scanning helps us recognize the signs of stress buildup. Fortunately, some of these signs are easily detected; for example, there is the pounding heart rate, the pressure in the head, the rapid breathing, and the taut muscles.

One of the best forms of body scanning is the monitoring of the condition of our muscles. Tense, overworked muscles accumulate lactic acid, a residue of neuronal firing in the muscle tissue. Neuronal firing is analogous to the firing of compressed gases in the compression chamber of an automobile cylinder. Both require the proper admixture of fuels. If the automatic choke on an automobile malfunctions (the butterfly valve remains closed), the air supply to the carburetor is cut off, and the automobile runs on pure gasoline vapor. Carbon then builds up in the carburetor, combustion chambers, and valves, and the engine stutters and spurts. Similarly, an abnormal buildup of lactic acid occurs in the body if the ratio of oxygen to organic fuel is disturbed. When under stress, this ratio is disturbed, and lactic acid builds up at a faster-than-normal rate.

Lactic acid fatigues muscle tissue and brings on the feeling of anxiety. The greater the amount of lactic acid, the more intense is the experience of anxiety. Indeed, calm people can be made to feel anxious with an injection of lactic acid.[2]

If we learn to monitor the early buildup of stress, we can prevent its spiraling effects. The key is early detection, and the prime focus should be on the muscles. Once muscular tension has built to disastrous levels, it is difficult to lower it. We can successfully counter the tension with relaxation methods, however, if it is recognized early.

## Seek Information Regarding the Stressor

The natural tendency in facing stressful situations is to ignore them. It is as though we believe that they will go away if we look the other way.

While it may be wise to tolerate rather than to combat stressors at times, it would be unwise to do so without carefully assessing them first. Reticent, nonassertive people often tolerate stressors that could be eliminated economically.

First, review what you already know about the stressor. Be mindful that your native inclination is to magnify its seriousness. Ask yourself, "What is really happening?" Strive for a more objective view of the stressor. You may find that your stress derives more from a resentment of having to use your time and energy than from fear of being unable to handle the stressor. Make associations between this situation and others you have handled successfully.

Next, ask others about the situation. Use networking in dealing with it. Who do you know that has dealt with this situation before? What can they tell you about it? Can they tell you the best way of handling it? Stressful situations often are so upsetting that we take action before seeking vital information. We seek relief so desperately that we take precipitous action. Getting the facts often proves stress-reducing as situations are seldom as bad as our imagination represents them as being.

Rehearse the worst-case scenario. Ask yourself, "What will happen if I don't cope successfully with this situation, and how bad will this be?" If you can remain objective in answering these questions, you may find that you could live with the consequences of the worst probable outcome. The consequences might not be desirable, but you could live with them. If you pass this test, you may reduce any panic the stressor might induce.

## Inventory Resources

Once the stressor has been engaged, it is important to take stock of your resources for coping with it. Most persons underestimate their resources. Because the body does not know the difference between fact and fantasy, it braces itself for an onslaught when you predict failure. A more objective appraisal of your resources will significantly decrease your stress. Albert Bandura concluded that a sense of personal resourcefulness (efficacy) is the single most effective buffer against stress.[3] Because stress often results from perceiving demands to be greater than resources, a more generous appraisal of resources will counter the tendency to "catastrophize" and thus reduce the stress.

# Establishing Detente or Waging War

Once we have accurately appraised demands and resources, we must decide whether to coexist with the stressor or to declare war on it. It is not always easy to make this decision. While it is wasteful to fight unnecessary battles, it is also wasteful to adjust to stressors that could be eliminated with decisive action. The importance of wasting energy becomes underlined if we accept Selye's concept of limited adaptation energy.[4]

Selye maintained that each of us inherits a *limited* quantity of energy with which to adapt to stressors. This energy is nonreplenishable. Indeed, aging is the process of using up this energy. The more wasteful we are with our supply, the faster we age. Consequently, the proper management of this limited adaptation energy is a matter of life or death.

Selye held that some of this energy was readily available while some was held in reserve. If all readily available energy were to be used up before the reserve energy could be mobilized, the organism would die without having exhausted its reserve supply. Exhibit 4–1 draws upon a historical event to depict this relationship.

On 1 September 1939, Nazi Germany shamelessly unleashed its war machine on Poland without warning. The genius of the German military strategy was called *blitzkrieg,* which meant lightning-like war. The Luftwaffe rained metal terror from the skies. The troops of the Wehrmacht behind the mechanized panzer divisions violated Polish borders from three directions. Simultaneously the German fifth column created political havoc in the major Polish cities. These sudden multifaceted attacks quickly exhausted Poland's standing army and it was forced to capitulate.

Historians have since concluded that Poland alone may have been a match for the Nazis had it had time to mobilize its reserves. Ironically, Hitler placed his troops in the same untenable position by inviting conflict on all borders of the German state. Under these conditions even Germany's ablest military strategists were unable to save the country from defeat.

## Establishing Detente

At times it is best to make peace with our challengers, to live *with* the burr under the saddle, to save our energy for more important battles. There is nothing cowardly about tolerating irritants if the cost of remov-

**Exhibit 4-1.** Blitzkrieg: The Sudden Exhaustion of Adaptation Energy

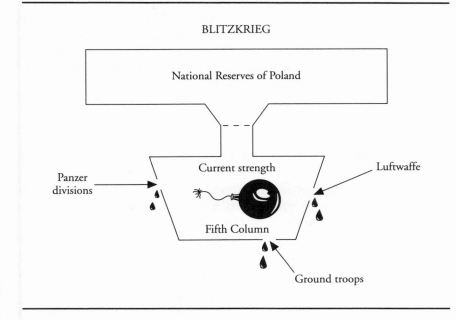

ing them is too great. If, however, we tolerate stressors because we do not trust our resources, the price in the long run may be enormous! As pointed out in chapter 2, Michael Antoni referred to this adjustment as a passive form of coping that inhibits the immune system and renders us vulnerable to cancer and infectious diseases.[5]

In deciding whether to adjust to the stressor or to try to eliminate it, ask yourself "Can I do anything about it?" If the answer is "No," the issue is decided. You *must* adjust to it. If the answer is "Yes," ask yourself a second question: "Am I *willing* to do anything about it?" Again, if the answer is "No," you must choose detente. There are many situations in which we can take action but may choose not to do so. We may believe that removing the stressor would be too costly, and, there-fore, it would be best to tolerate it.

Events that we cannot or will not change should be reframed. Reframing is a matter of viewing events from a different perspective in order to change their meaning. Emotional reactions to events are largely deter-mined by the meanings we assign them. The assigning of meaning is a very subjective matter. Quite often we do not have enough facts to be certain of the interpretations we make. Most events allow for a number of competing interpretations, and each of these interpretations may lead to a different emotional reaction. The other side of every liability is an asset. Generally, there is something redeeming about every situation if we look for it. This idea is nicely captured in the Chinese definition of crisis as offering both danger *and* opportunity. The reframe should not be a hype; it must be at *least* as likely as the old frame if it is to be effective.

Most of us have had experiences that seemed at the time most unfortunate, only to find later that they led to valuable outcomes. When a spouse divorces you, you may see the event as being an unmitigated disaster. When, you have had time to readjust, however, you may wish to thank your spouse for having done you a favor. At least, now you have the freedom to redefine yourself. Mel Kranzler discussed these salutary options in *The Creative Divorce.*[6] Obviously, stressors such as divorce do not always come to such happy ends. But in part the result depends on the manner in which you frame it. At times you may need to be quite creative in constructing reframes. One promising tact is to ask yourself "What can I learn from this situation?"

A client of one of the authors has recently undergone a series of shocking blows to her security. The father of her two small children defaulted on his child support. A restructuring of her corporation resulted in a significant loss of income. Her preschool son was diagnosed as having an attention deficit disorder and was in need of expensive medication. And her recently estranged boyfriend called to tell her he had tested positive for the AIDS virus. All of these developments occurred within a span of two weeks.

Prior to these stressful developments, she had been making considerable progress in adopting a more positive view of herself and others. Obviously, such developments occasioned a temporary relapse. Once we had exhausted all the real-life options she had for dealing with her situation, we attempted to reframe the situation. We struggled to see these developments as offering a unique laboratory for using her newly learned reframing skills. We were both aware that the rate of her progress would increase astronomically if she were able to chart a steady course at the time, and to use these threats to her security as a cue to practice her relaxation skills and positive affirmations. While all of the necessary adjustments have not yet been completed, she is dealing functionally with them at the present *and* is coming to view her coping resources as being considerably more adequate than she had thought.

She has successfully reframed this potentially disastrous situation as an opportunity for rapid personal growth.

## Waging War

We should calculate the cost before we decide to attack the stressor. If we emotionally accept the costs *before* we declare war on the stressor, we will escape the additional stress that we experience when we meet unanticipated costs. The kind of resolve that works best is one that includes a great deal of patience. Realizing that the battle will be difficult and costly will prepare us for the duress and tediousness of the commitment.

Many persons focus their attention on the management of their emotions when confronting stressors. Focusing *mostly* on one's emotions usually makes things worse. For anxious reactive persons, awareness of anxious symptoms cues additional arousal. The energy tied up in this manner limits the amount left to be directed to the stressor. Meichenbaum's Stress Inoculation technique teaches the client to reframe these symptoms as cues for initiating a planned attack on the stressor.[7] The planned attack calls for elaborate efforts to keep one's attention clearly focused on the *task* at hand rather than on one's emotions.

# Watch Your Thinking in Stressful Situations

Much stress is self-generated. We are constantly carrying on one-way conversations with ourselves about the meaning of our experience. This self-talk is strongly influenced by our beliefs about ourselves, the world, and ourselves in relation to the world. In one of the passages from Carlos Castaneda's *A Separate Reality,* Don Juan says:

> The world is such-and-such or so-and-so only because we tell ourselves that is the way it is . . . You talk to yourself. You're not unique at that. Every one of us does that. We carry on internal talk . . . In fact we maintain our world with our internal talk.[8]

Many current therapies emphasize the importance of beliefs in determining stress levels. The Individual Psychology of Alfred Adler, the Rational Emotive Therapy of Albert Ellis, the Transactional Analysis of Berne, and cognitive-behaviorists all emphasize the crucial role played by beliefs in creating stressful emotions.

The idea that behavior can be changed by thought control is hardly new. It has been stated time and again in the world's great literature.

Shakespeare has Hamlet say: "There is nothing either good or bad but thinking makes it so." In the Old Testament we read, "As a man thinketh in his heart, so is he," and in the New Testament "Finally, brethren, whatsoever things are true. . . honest . . . just . . . pure . . . lovely . . . of good report; if there be any virtue, and if there be any praise, think on these things." Right thinking is one of the chief practices recommended by Buddhists for the good life. Faith in the importance of thinking as a guide to behavior underlies the practice of advertising, political brainwashing, and more legitimate forms of education.

Behavior is largely a function of expectations of future events. If we want to write poetry, try out for the varsity football team, or begin a business, and we believe we have no talent for such things, we probably will not try. Talent, of course, is important, but expectations frequently make the difference. Very often believing is *seeing*. Robert Rosenthal called this phenomenon the self-fulfilling prophecy.[9] If we tell ourselves convincingly that we are going to fail, this expectation is likely to become reality. A promising way of reducing the amount of stress with which we must cope is to replace nonfunctional self-talk with more *functional* self-talk. Many research studies in the sixties support the assumption that beliefs and their resulting self-talk influence emotions.

Stanley Schachter and Jerome Singer attempted to determine if the effects of situations contrived to bring about strong feeling would depend upon the explanations (beliefs) available to subjects. Three groups of subjects were given injections of epinephrine. Before being exposed to the contrived situations, one group was told of the true effects of epinephrine; a second group was given an inaccurate explanation; and the third group was given no explanation. In each situation the group that was properly informed of the effects of epinephrine were less influenced by the contrived situations than were other groups. The informed group members believed that their arousal was a direct result of the epinephrine, while the other groups attributed their arousal to the contrived situations. These latter groups reported greater emotional responses to the contrived situations than did the informed group.[10]

Robert Nisbett and Stanley Schachter gave their subjects a placebo and then subjected them to mild electrical shock. Half of their subjects were told that their emotional arousal following the shock was largely a result of the properties of the pill. Subsequently, these subjects tolerated four times more shock than other subjects. Expectations arising from their beliefs appeared to influence strongly the amount of emotional duress they tolerated.[11]

Velton asked his subjects to read statements selected for their presumed ability to elicit certain emotional responses. One group read "elated" statements, another "depressed" statements, and yet another "neutral" statements. He presumed that the emotional effects of reading these statements would have differential effects on their subsequent performances on several behavioral tasks. On the majority of these tasks, the "elated" group outperformed the other two.[12]

In a similar study Rimm and Litvak found that subjects who read emotionally loaded statements registered greater arousal on standard physiological measures than did subjects reading emotionally neutral statements. Words are powerful stimulants to emotions. The choice of words used to label experiences is important. If we explain our reactions with labels such as "hopping mad" or "scared to death," we are more likely to increase physiological arousal than if we use labels such as "irritated" or "excited." The important thing, of course, is that the explanation must be believable.[13]

## Checking the Logic of Self-talk

Most people assume that emotional reactions are a direct response to some unpleasant situation. We are angry *because* the mechanic failed to properly repair our automobile, or we are afraid *because* we must speak before a class. We talk as though the mechanic and the class have the power to cause us to be angry or fearful.

In reality such things do not cause anger or fear; rather, we cause ourselves to become angry or fearful by what we say to ourselves about these events. We make one or more faulty assumptions about why things happen, and these assumption lead us in unrewarding directions. Voltaire said "Madness is having incorrect perceptions and reasoning correctly from them." In the case of the mechanic, we might say, "Darn him, I doubt that he even touched those brakes. Probably just left the car in the stall for a couple of hours and then turned the ticket in to the cashier as though the repair had been made." This anger, then, is a function of *attributing* the mechanic's behavior to malevolent intentions, believing that we were purposely exploited. Similarly, the fear of addressing the class is a function of what we are saying to ourselves about the class's response. When we say something like "I'm going to make a fool out of myself. I'm not going to be able to remember a thing, and they are going to make fun of me," it is not the group, but our *thoughts* that make us fearful.

Usually there are alternative explanations for these events that will lead to different emotional responses. Of the mechanic's failure we could have said, "It's an honest mistake. He was probably pushed for time and, without knowing it, failed to complete the repair." And of the class we could have said, "They know how it is; their turn is coming. They are probably pulling for me." These alternate beliefs would undoubtedly lead to less stressful reactions. The following summarizes the relationship between events, self-talk, and emotional response.

$$\text{Actual event} \longrightarrow \text{Explanation to self} \longrightarrow \text{Physiological response} \longrightarrow \text{Emotional label}$$

The labeling of emotional responses does not follow directly from an actual event. The key to the situation appears to be the intervening self-talk, the explanation that we give ourselves of the event. This explanation results in an emotional label that causes the physiological arousal. The following shows the emotional responses in the case of the mechanic and the class speech:

**Mechanic's failure**   "Exploitation"⟶ Strong arousal⟶ Anger

"Honest mistake"⟶ Mild arousal⟶ Disappointment

**Speaking before class**   "They'll make fun" ⟶ Strong arousal ⟶ Panic

"They're pulling ⟶ Mild arousal ⟶ Concern for me"

When we realize that our emotional reactions follow directly from our beliefs and self-talk, we can no longer escape responsibility for our emotional reactions. We then realize that it is our choice whether to become disturbed over events or take them in our stride. The criticism of others, for instance, can hurt us only if we let it.

Thus, we can change our emotional reactions by changing our perceptions of events. Although we might say of someone who stares at us in a puzzling manner, "He makes me so angry when he looks at me with that silly smirk on his face," this angry response is not actually a reaction to the facial expression, but rather, a reaction to the explanation we give ourselves for his facial expression. The emotional response would be quite different if we adopted the following explanation, "He reacts with a silly smile because he's embarrassed by his inability to think of an appropriate comeback, and his smile is his only defense." We will feel a great deal more control if we realize that the key to our emotions resides in our heads, not in the actions of others.

## The Unholy Trilogy of Beliefs

Albert Ellis suggests that people choose hurtful explanations for events because they have adopted certain nonfunctional beliefs from society. He believes such nonfunctional beliefs account for much of the neurosis of our times. He lists a trilogy of nonfunctional beliefs that he believes are widely prevalent in American culture:

1. I *should* be perfectly competent and masterful, and I am a *worthless* individual if I am not.
2. Others *should* treat me considerately and fairly, and if they don't, they are rotten people.
3. The world *should* arrange for me to experience pleasure rather than pain, and life is horrible and I *can't bear it* if the world doesn't.[14]

Ellis maintains that these irrational ideas lead to emotional disturbance because they cannot be lived up to successfully. He wrote:

> Once a human being believes the kind of nonsense included in these notions, he will inevitably tend to become inhibited, hostile, defensive, guilty, ineffective, inert, uncontrolled, unhappy. If, on the other hand, he could become thoroughly released from all these fundamental kinds of illogical thinking, it would be exceptionally difficult for him to become intensely emotionally upset, or at least to sustain his disturbance for any extended period.[15]

Since the explanations for things that happen are often determined by such nonfunctional beliefs, we often turn ordinary experiences into significant stressors. These faulty editorials about events in our lives trigger strong emotions. If we can ferret out these culprits—these faulty editorials—and exchange them for more reasonable ones, we can greatly reduce the stress and misery in our lives. Aaron Beck focuses on distorted cognitive processes, that is, dysfunctional ways persons process information about themselves and their environment.[16] With a little detective work, anyone can begin to spot the irrationality in thought processes. The following thinking distortions are adapted from Beck.

*Blow-up.* Many people have a tendency to exaggerate the seriousness of an event all out of proportion to the actual situation. Such a tendency toward overgeneralization can lead people to conclude that they will never do anything right after making a single mistake. Blow-up thinking can also lead to statements such as, "Uncle Edward hasn't answered my letter. I just know he hates me" or "Jack's a big snob. He didn't come over to speak with me after the meeting." In such cases we take small bits of information and assign enormous importance to them. In so doing, we often make unjustifiable jumps in logic and draw conclusions from evidence that is either lacking or actually contrary to the conclusion reached. This logical error stems from creating general rules from single incidents.

*All-or-nothing Thinking.* This is a kind of polarized thinking in which people think in extremes; for example, interpreting a mild rebuff as a total rejection. In these cases only two possibilities are allowed: right or wrong, good or bad, always or never, all or nothing. We say things such as, "I *always* mess up on exams" or "People *never* have a good time with me." Such dichotomous thinking obscures the many shades of opinion made possible by more discriminating thinking. If we say, "People *sometimes* seem to be bored with my company," then we can begin to examine the differences in our behavior in those situations in which others are bored verses those in which they are not. Then we may choose whether or not we wish to behave in a way that will interest them. This kind of discriminating thinking often leads to more functional outcomes than does all-or-nothing thinking.

*Personalization.* With this kind of thinking persons incorrectly assume responsibility for external events, for example, allowing oneself to feel responsible for the behavior of a grown son or daughter.

*Projective Thinking.* Projective thinking is the opposite of personalization. Here people project the responsibility for their emotions and personal worth onto others. They say, "He makes me so angry I can't stand it!" or "I would be a more stable person today if my father hadn't been such a drunkard." They project the responsibility onto others because they wish to escape responsibility for their own behavior. In the first example it is easier to blame the other person for our anger than it is to recognize that *we* are making ourselves angry by the meaning we assign to his behavior. In the second example we make use of a favorite villain—in this case it happens to be the father.

*Perfectionistic Thinking.* People sometimes demonstrate a brittle kind of perfectionism in their thinking. Nothing short of a perfect performance is worthwhile. Such an attitude is exemplified by comments such as, "So what if I got an A. It was barely over the line" or "Being second may be good enough for Avis, but let me tell you, nobody worth his salt will settle for coming in second."

*Selective Abstraction.* Here the person attends to a detail while ignoring the context; for example, focusing on the failure of your spouse to show keen interest in your conversation, you interpret the behavior as a slight without noticing that he or she is deeply worried about the family's finances.

*Self-punishing Thinking.* Sometimes we become so disappointed with ourselves that we lose sight of the task. We mope around while opportunities for improvement pass us by. This self-punishing thinking results in a poor self-image, which in turn makes failure more likely. Statements such as, "I usually don't remember names, so there is really no use in trying to do so" or "I'm so dumb . . . that's the third straight shot I've missed" are clues to this attitude. Anything that diverts attention from the task is likely to be self-defeating, and self-punishing thoughts certainly do so.

## Correcting Self-talk

What we say to ourselves about our abilities at the time we are combating stressors strongly influences the degree of stress we shall experience. Indeed, Deal and Williams found these immediate negative cognitions (self-talk) to be more predictive of depression than measures of irrational beliefs or dysfunctional attitudes.[17] We can learn about our own self-talk problems by attempting to identify traces of dysfunctionality in others. Study the examples in Exhibit 4–2. First, decide whether or not the statement is dysfunctional. If so, then decide whether it is an example of blow-up, all-or-nothing thinking, personalization, projective thinking, perfectionist thinking, selective abstraction, or self-punishing thinking. The answers are listed at the end of the chapter.

Obviously, the most important thing is to be able to discriminate between functional and nonfunctional self-sentences. Consequently your score in the No/Yes column is considerably more important than your score in the Type column. (In fact, the types often have two or more suitable answers.) After scoring the answers with the help of the scoring key, consult the interpretive key also at the end of the chapter.

**Exhibit 4–2.** Identifying Dysfunctional Self-talk

| NO | YES | | TYPE |
|---|---|---|---|
| ___ | ___ | 1. OK, so I don't always get A's; but that doesn't mean I'm stupid. | ___ |
| ___ | ___ | 2. I'm so stupid. No wonder people hate me. | ___ |
| ___ | ___ | 3. Mr. Smith doesn't like me because he allows others to offer their financial analyses before he asks for mine. | ___ |
| ___ | ___ | 4. Darn it, the cake fell. Guess I'd better read the instructions next time. | ___ |
| ___ | ___ | 5. I'm doing it again! I always talk too much every single time I meet somebody. | ___ |
| ___ | ___ | 6. June turned me down. That's disappointing, but there are other girls I can ask out. | ___ |
| ___ | ___ | 7. John hasn't called me from the convention yet. I can image how pressured he is by that committee assignment. | ___ |
| ___ | ___ | 8. If I had been a better mother, Sheldon would have been a more responsible person. | ___ |
| ___ | ___ | 9. If I can't clear up every single blemish, then there's no way I'm going to that wedding. | ___ |
| ___ | ___ | 10. That proves it! I won't be able to pass any of those tests no matter how long I study. | ___ |
| ___ | ___ | 11. Unless I can work out every detail, I'll never offer another proposal to my boss. | ___ |
| ___ | ___ | 12. I never make a good first impression. So I might as well prepare myself for rejection. | ___ |
| ___ | ___ | 13. He's made me so upset there's no way I'm going to be able to play decent tennis. | ___ |
| ___ | ___ | 14. I don't care if he was in the last game of the tennis match, he should have noticed that I was tired and wanted to go home. | ___ |
| ___ | ___ | 15. Whoops! Missed that shot, but then my average is pretty good so far. | ___ |

## Steps For Correcting Stressful Self-talk

The following steps for dealing with self-talk may prove useful:

1. When experiencing stress, listen to the internal monologue. If you cannot "hear" yourself saying the words, ask, "What *could* I be saying to myself that would account for my emotional response."

2. Decide whether or not your self-talk explanation is nonfunc-

tional in one or more of the previously mentioned ways; that is, does the explanation make use of blow-up, all-or-nothing thinking, personalization, projective thinking, perfectionist thinking, selective abstraction, or self-punishing thinking?

3. Take a second look at the actual situation, just the specifics, never mind the interpretation or explanation. Strive for a more objective understanding of what *actually* happened.

4. Generate alternative explanations for the actual situation. Do not suggest highly unlikely explanations. These alternatives must be at least as likely as the one causing you distress at the moment.

5. Review these alternative explanations. For each of the alternatives ask yourself "If I accepted this alternative explanation, how would I feel?"

6. Because all of the alternatives should represent believable explanations for the situation, and since each leads to a differing emotional response on your part, remind yourself that you can choose how you wish to feel by your choice of an alternative.

7. Choose a more functional explanation from among these alternatives and begin to operate on the basis of it.

8. Attempt to convince others of the relationship between their faulty self-talk and their emotional responses (but do it delicately!). One of the best ways of learning is to teach others.

Let us apply these steps to the following common experience. Bill has just received a test score from one of his instructors, and his reaction is highly self-punishing: "I flunked the damned exam! How stupid! No one who is as dumb as I am ought to be going to college anyway. Maybe I had better hang it up." This kind of talk is nonfunctional. It does not suggest constructive actions, and it is disheartening. This is clearly an example of Blow-up. The results of one examination led Bill to conclude that he was stupid, dumb, and unable to measure up in college. Moreover, he also engaged in Self-punishing Thinking. All this talk about being stupid and dumb misdirects his attention from the task. Such talk is unlikely to lead to constructive action but is likely to injure his self image.

Taking a second, more objective, look at the situation may suggest that Bill did *not* flunk the test at all. Sometimes a grade such as 75 or 80 is taken as failure, provided one's self-expectations are extremely high. Perhaps Bill would conclude, on second look, that, in reality, he had made a C or B, and while this is below his expectations, it is hardly a failing grade.

Alternative explanations for his performance actually may be more reasonable than the one Bill had given himself. Perhaps it is not that he is "dumb," but that the exam was poorly written, or the instructor used an old and inappropriate examination. Or perhaps Bill did not study enough, or did not study the right topics. These alternative explanations will lead to different emotional responses. If he chooses to believe that the exam was poorly written, he may turn self-deprecation into irritation toward the instructor for his slipshod work. If he chooses to believe that he had studied too little or inappropriately, then he can talk with others to see what he should have studied. This alternative may prove more helpful in coping with similar situations in the future than either of the others. After identifying alternative explanations, Bill should select the more promising of these and to begin to take appropriate action.

In summary, irrational thinking creates a great deal of unnecessary stress. The process for eliminating such thinking involves taking a more realistic look at the troublesome situation, generating alternative explanations that are equally as likely as the explanation of the situation creating the stress, and taking action based on an alternative that leads to a constructive outcome and positive emotional response.

## Stress Inoculation

Meichenbaum devised an approach to stress control, which he calls stress inoculation.[18] He maintains that we guide our behavior with covert instructions and that, quite frequently, these instructions militate against our best adjustment. When meeting stressful situations, we often self-destruct by predicting failure. We are apt to think fear-inducing thoughts such as "Oh, no! I can't do it. Why do I let myself in for things like this?" These instructions are like tapes that automatically turn on inside our heads each time we encounter a certain type of stressful situation. They are so routine that we usually are unaware that they are running. Once habituated, these tapes lead to a general sense of helplessness when we encounter the stressor. Stress inoculation is designed to move us from a sense of learned helplessness to a sense of learned resourcefulness.

Each time we experience a new situation we give ourselves instructions for coping with it. The first few times we repeat the instructions aloud. One of the authors noticed his son instructing himself aloud when he was first learning to drive. He whispered the following directions to himself: "Let's see, I put the key in the ignition, put my foot on the clutch. The gear is in neutral. Turn the key, and now give it a little gas." These audible instructions soon become inaudible and embedded in our unconscious.

When we become stressed, our attention wanders from the task at hand and focuses on symptoms of arousal. We become aware of increasing tension and often say things to ourselves that increase the stress. A self-defeating cycle develops in which the more stressed we become, the more stress-engendering and nonfunctional are our self-instructions, and the more nonfunctional the self-instructions, the greater the failure and resulting stress.

With stress inoculation we learn to use the arousal cues (increased heart rate, flushed face, and the like) as triggers to recite functional self-instructions that are to replace self-defeating ones. The new self-instructions move the focus away from the arousal itself and toward task orientation. Essentially we say, "I feel myself getting anxious. I'm glad I recognized it early because if I begin my program for coping now, I can handle this situation. Now, let's see, just exactly what is it that I should be doing?" Such reassuring self-talk, however, is of little value unless we have a well-developed coping plan in mind.

Functional self-instructions accomplish four purposes: (1) they replace anxiety-engendering ones; (2) they lower arousal; (3) they direct attention to the relevant dimensions of the task; and (4) they encourage us to endorse ourselves for having managed the stressful situation. The forms of self-instruction typically used in stress inoculation follow.

## Instructions to Relax

Arousal cues are to remind us to begin the plan by relaxing. Since we ordinarily do not have a great deal of time to prepare for stressors, a prescribed breathing technique (to be discussed later in this chapter) is the preferred method of relaxing for this technique. At this point the self-instructions may go something like this: "Okay, I see I'm getting anxious, so it's time for my controlled breathing."

## Instructions to Remain Task-relevant

After relaxing we are to turn our attention to the specifics of the task. If we are taking an examination, the self-instruction may go something like this: "The breathing is helping a bit, so now I'm ready to look at the task. What is this question asking? What are the options? Let's see, I'm first to eliminate the options that clearly are incorrect. Okay, now which of these remaining options seem most likely?"

Stress inoculation anticipates potential relapse situations and prepares self-instructions beforehand to deal with them. For example, persons with examination anxiety may remember that they sometimes panic when they see other students finishing quickly. To handle this crisis they may instruct themselves to remain calm and say, "It's not important how quickly others finish. I have plenty of time. It won't make any difference to my grade if every student finishes before me." If they tend to panic when they are unable to remember some answer, they might say to themselves "I can't expect myself to be able to dredge up all facts instantaneously on cue. I will just check this question and come back to it. In the meantime I may see something in another question that will remind me of the answer to this question. Now, I just need to pause when I'm getting anxious like this and focus my attention solely on the question. I won't focus on my nervous symptoms as that would only make things worse."

Self-instructions may take widely varying forms, depending on the task. The important thing is to have some meaningful structure with which to combat anxiety. Structure, almost any structure, helps counter the helplessness that turns fear into panic. The most important self-instructions are those encouraging task relevancy.

## Instructions to Endorse Oneself

What we say to ourselves about newly acquired behaviors largely determines whether or not they are maintained. It is important to endorse ourselves after we have used our new self-instructions. We might say something like "Okay, I did it! I managed to go through the scene with my full attention on the task. I consciously directed my attention. I didn't remain helplessly adrift in all that anxiety. From here on out things should get better."

These instructions may seem naive to some readers. Indeed, they almost seem too simple to work. Still, many people have found them to be helpful in countering the self-defeating scripts they have recited for years. *At the least*, the new script will divert their attention from old anxiety engendering ones. As they practice these self-instruction in stress-inducing situations, they are apt to gain confidence in their ability to cope with these situations.

## Symptom Prescription

Paradoxically, help sometimes consists of prescribing the very behavior that causes our stress. Dunlap prescribed stuttering for stutterers in order to help them bring the habit under conscious control.[19] This technique is one of the primary ways speech therapists work with stutterers. The use of this technique assumes that fear of committing the behavior is the chief cause of the behavior itself. Hence, if a person can bring a behavior under conscious control, the automatic nature of the behavior is destroyed. Stutterers may be instructed to practice stuttering while purchasing items in a department store, while talking on the telephone, or while speaking in class. If they can will themselves to stutter, so the argument goes, they can will themselves to stop stuttering.

Symptom prescription has been used with people suffering other involuntary stress symptoms. One of the authors used the technique with an impotent husband. His impotency stemmed from fear that he would be unable to have an erection. The couple was instructed to freely engage in sensate focusing, that is, activities such as showering together or massaging each other, activities that had been sexually arousing earlier in their marriage. But under no circumstance were they to engage in intercourse during the week. The couple smiled and agreed to the prescription. The following week they sheepishly confessed that they had been unable to keep the contract. Prohibiting them from having intercourse had lowered the husband's anxiety, and the prescribed playful activities had aroused him sufficiently to perform. He was aware that he could cite the therapist's prohibition against intercourse as an acceptable excuse were he unable to have an erection. The pressure was relieved, and he was able to respond normally.

Symptom prescription is sometimes used with perfectionists who are deathly afraid of making mistakes. Secretaries are asked to make small mistakes on purpose. Ball players are asked to drop passes, to strike out, or to miss shots. Great care is exercised, however, to insure that such mistakes are not likely to become catastrophes. Purposefully making small, unimportant errors sometimes helps persons to discover that the consequences of failure are not as great as believed. Fear of making mistakes is often incapacitating, and symptom prescription can help to lessen its grip.

Victor Frankl uses a form of symptom prescription that he calls paradoxical intention.[20] It involves a deliberate attempt to evoke humor in regard to a troublesome behavior. The client is encouraged to deliberately exaggerate a symptom. If the client is afraid of blushing, he is told to turn ever redder and redder until his face is fire-engine red. If he is afraid of sweating profusely in public, he is told to sweat torrents of perspiration that will drench everything in sight. If he is afraid of stumbling through a speech, he is told to stumble deliberately as much as he can. He is to imagine the audience booing, grimacing, and laughing raucously at his expense. He is to further imagine the news wires and television networks reporting his stumbling performance to a national audience, to imagine his performance being discussed on the floor of the General Assembly of the United Nations, and so on, *ad absurdium*. The humor of the exaggerated embarrassment is often enough to defuse a situation of its anxiety-arousing potential.

## Cooling Down the Human Machine

Hyperarousal generally interferes with effective coping. Any comprehensive approach to stress management must include relaxation procedures. Some relaxation procedures are more appropriate for emergency conditions. Some take too much time for an emergency but have more powerful effects.

### Emergency Techniques

Emergency relaxation techniques are useful when one does not have much time to prepare for stressful situations. Having to confront a subordinate, to ask the boss for a raise, or having to give a speech are all situations in which a short relaxation procedure would be quite useful. Two such procedures are Prescribed Breathing and the Quieting Response.

*Prescribed Breathing.* One of the quickest ways of reducing heightened physiological arousal is through proper breathing. Our breathing becomes dysrhythmic when we are stressed. A few minutes of regulated breathing often will reduce arousal and help us to think more precisely. The effects of prescribed breathing will not last for long but will help nicely in those tense situations that bring on immobilizing anxiety. For example, we may freeze in our supervisor's office when trying to share a new idea. Or we may sense that a discussion is approaching a serious confrontation and become overwhelmed by strong emotion. In such situations, it is important to remain calm, to use one's faculties without suffering the inhibiting effects of anxiety.

Quite often we are able to manage our anxiety rather well if we can get into the stressful situation in a calm manner. By remaining calm early on we can create a reaction in others that puts us at ease. If feedback from others in these first few critical moments suggests that our performance is appropriate and well-received, it is easier for us to maintain composure throughout. Very often, then, what is needed is merely a temporary kind of control over anxiety. For this purpose, the prescribed breathing technique seems ideal.

Stress disturbs the natural breathing rhythm. We may breathe rapidly and shallowly and thus bring on hyperventilation, or we may breathe too slowly and inefficiently, setting up a condition known as hypoxia. In both cases the resulting feeling is distress. Prescribed breathing reduces stress through a perfectly balanced breathing ratio, expressed as 3–12–6. That is, take 3 seconds for inhaling, 12 seconds for holding the breath, and 6 seconds for exhaling.

We should prepare for these breathing exercises by sitting comfortably with feet firmly planted on the floor, body weight evenly distributed along the spine, eyes closed, and tight garments appropriately loosened. Run through six cycles of the 3–12–6 breathing. Then let your breathing return to normal. Sit for a couple minutes more, and each time you breathe out visualize your body collapsing and sinking further and further into the seat of your chair. The feeling of heaviness accompanies profound relaxation; therefore, inducing the feeling with your imagination will further the natural relaxation from regulated breathing. Practice this exercise daily and your confidence in its effectiveness will increase. If begun early in the stress cycle, a couple minutes of such breathing will bring noticeable relief.

*Quieting Response.* Martin Ford et al. suggest a visualization approach for relaxation.[21] One is to say "Alert mind, calm body" and then smile inwardly. Do it slowly and visualize the muscles throughout your body loosening as you say "calm body". Allow the inward smile to develop fully in your imagination while paying particular attention to the relaxing of muscles in the jaw and cheek area. Recent studies by ethologists confirm the observation of Darwin that the act of smiling effectively alters the mood state.[22] Inhale slowly imagining that the breath is coming from your feet. Exhale the same way. Sense a wave of warmth and heaviness coming over you. Let your shoulders slump.

## More Powerful Techniques

The following techniques are considerably more effective in inducing a profound state of relaxation; however, they require considerably more time. Four techniques to be given special attention are Deep Muscle Relaxation, the Relaxation Response, Alpha Training, and aerobic exercise.

*Deep Muscle Relaxation.* When stressed, the muscles contract strongly. The result is the feeling of tension. With chronic stress the muscles may contract so long that they begin to spasm, bringing on pain. There is a direct positive feedback loop between the neurons embedded in muscles and the hypothalamus. When muscles begin to tense, these neurons inform the hypothalamus and it in turn intensifies the tightening. On the other hand, when the muscles begin to loosen, these neurons likewise inform the hypothalamus, and it now facilitates the loosening. One can relax the muscles directly by mental control or calm the mind by loosening the muscles. It works both ways. With the deep muscle relaxation technique one seeks to calm the mind by relaxing the muscles.

This technique will be more effective if you are properly prepared. Use a comfortable, padded chair. Sit upright, but not rigidly. Let the weight of the body rest solidly upon the spine. Do not cross arms or legs. Remove such constraining items as watches, rings, eyeglasses, contact lenses, and shoes. Loosen ties and unbutton collars. Seek a quiet, dimly lit place where you can be alone. The steps involved in deep-muscle relaxation are simple. Move systematically through the thirteen muscle groups listed in Exhibit 4–3. Tense a muscle for 7 seconds, then relax it for 20–30 seconds before going on the next muscle. The entire routine will take between 15–20 minutes.

There are two reasons for tensing muscles before attempting to relax them. First, it is important to learn the feeling of a tense muscle in order to be able to detect tension early in the stress cycle. Tensing a muscle for a few seconds and studying the feeling of tension is excellent practice for monitoring stress symptoms. You will be able to begin self-treatment before the tension builds to excessive levels if you recognize it in the early stages. Second, the muscle will lengthen more if it has first been contracted. The effect is analogous to lifting the pendulum of a clock to its maximum height on one side, then allowing it to swing completely

**Exhibit 4-3.** Muscle Groups for Deep Muscle Relaxation

---

1.  Extend the arms and clench the fist to the point of pressure but not pain.
2.  Extend the arms again and imaginarily push a wall out there by extending the fingers toward the ceiling.
3.  Extend the arms sideways and then bend at the elbow, touching the shoulders with the tips of the fingers.
4.  Shut your eyes tightly (if you are not wearing contact lenses) and create pressure over the scalp, in the forehead and temples, and around the eyes.
5.  Push your tongue up against the palate, chomp down on your molar teeth, and bring the corners of your lips back around toward your ears.
6.  Bring your chin down approximately one inch off the sternum bone and attempt to do the impossible—that is pull the head down and back at the *same* time. This will set up great pressure in the neck muscles.
7.  Take a deep breath and scrunch the shoulders up toward the ears.
8.  Take another deep breath and try to touch the shoulders together in the back.
9.  Suck the stomach in, trying to touch the backbone with it.
10. Push the buttocks down into the seat of the chair.
11. Lift the heels off the floor about six inches to tense the thigh muscles.
12. Lift the heels again, pointing the toes toward the knees causing the shin muscles to contract and the calf muscles to stretch.
13. Lift the heels a third time, curling the toes toward the arch muscles.

---

to the opposite side upon its release. A contracted muscle relaxes more fully if it is first tensed.

Study the sources of pressure while tensing the muscle. Release the muscle all at once. It is sometimes helpful to hold your breath while tensing the muscle and then to release the breath and muscle together. There should be a sudden surge of relaxation, lasting one to two seconds. Study this feeling of relaxation also. Notice the difference between the feeling of tensed and relaxed muscles. Notice the feeling of warmth in the relaxed muscle. Each time you release a muscle visualize the muscle fibers making up the muscle spreading out and getting longer, looser, and more and more relaxed.

The desired effect is not limited to the surge of relaxation following the release of the tensed muscle, but rather to the sensation of deep relaxation that follows several minutes after its release. The muscle fibers continue to lengthen for several minutes after you have tensed the muscle. Go systematically from one muscle group to the next. After completing the routine mentally review each muscle. Imagine each of these muscles spreading out and becoming like cooked spaghetti. Sit for a few minutes longer just soaking up those warm feelings of deep muscle relaxation.

Certain outcomes of this practice are predictable. The body will feel heavier, the forehead will become cooler, and the palms warmer. Heartbeat and breathing rate will slow. Facial muscles may feel heavy. You may be reluctant to stir again since the sensation of relaxation will be so pleasant. Practicing these exercises on a daily basis will significantly lower your stress and raise your energy level. The extent of the help to be gained is directly related to the consistency with which the exercises are practiced.

*The Relaxation Response.* Nobel prize-winning physiologist Walter Hess discovered two centers within the brain that are associated with mutually incompatible emotional reactions. If the ergotropic center is triggered, the organism is prepared for fight or flight; if the trophotropic center is triggered, the organism experiences a high degree of relaxation. Herbert Benson, associate professor of medicine at Harvard, concluded that meditation triggers the trophotropic center and results in a sense of relaxation and well-being. He found that meditation activates, without side effects, a degree of muscular relaxation similar to that provided by tranquilizers. Herbert Benson calls this trophotropic reaction the *relaxation response* and has written about it in a book by the same title.[23]

Benson's technique is similar to Transcendental Meditation (TM). He studied similar practices found within the literature of psychology and religion and concluded that the effects of Transcendental Meditation, Zen and Yoga, autogenic training, progressive relaxation, hypnosis, and sentic cycles were all quite similar.

The relaxation response is a natural and innate protective mechanism that allows us to neutralize the harmful effects of excessive stress. It decreases heart rate, lowers metabolism, decreases rate of breathing, and brings the body back into a healthier balance. Consequently it is an effective antidote for the pervasive stress that is so much a part of modern living. Although Benson pieced together his technique mainly from the yogic forms of meditation, it is more likely to appeal to Westerners than the Eastern yogic forms because it is shorn of mystical elements and expressed in familiar terms. Moreover, the practice is supported by a large body of physiological research about oxygen consumption, respiratory rate, heartbeat, alpha waves, blood pressure, and muscle tension. Benson's research suggests that hypertension, migraine headaches, and addictive problems such as alcoholism and drug abuse are likely to be lessened by the regular use of the relaxation response.

**Exhibit 4-4.** Practicing the Relaxation Response

1. Sit quietly in a comfortable position with the eyes closed.
2. Relax deeply by imagining the muscles becoming looser, beginning with the feet and working up to the face.
3. Breathe easily and naturally through your nose. Each time you exhale silently repeat the word "one."
4. Continue the practice for ten to twenty minutes, and when finished, sit quietly for several minutes.
5. Maintain a passive attitude throughout. Do not try too hard. Ignore distracting thoughts and merely return to the rhythmic breathing and the repetition of the word "one" after each exhalation. Allow the relaxation to occur at its own pace.
6. Repeat this practice once or twice a day. Since the digestive processes appear to interfere with the relaxation response, allow two hours after any meal before beginning the practice.

*Source:* Herbert Benson, *The Relaxation Response* (New York: Morrow, 1975), 114–115.

The technique for inducing the relaxation response seems disarmingly simple. Indeed, there are some who might take it more seriously if it appeared to be more difficult. However, Benson's method is not quite as simple as it seems. It does require some persistence, but soon it will become second nature to the practitioner. The basic steps in inducing the relaxation response are listed in Exhibit 4-4.[24]

In his first book Benson was exclusively interested in the physiologic effects of the practice of meditation. However, in a later volume, *Beyond the Relaxation Response,* he emphasized the importance of what he called the "faith factor."[25] Over the years he came to appreciate the value of having users of the relaxation response choose mantras that had special spiritual significance for them. He suggested that persons of religious persuasion use part of a prayer or some sacred word instead of the word "one" that is typically used with the relaxation response. Catholics might use "Hail Mary, full of grace" or "Lord Jesus Christ, have mercy upon me." Jews might use the greeting, "Shalom," or the Hebrew word for one, "Echad!" Protestants might use the first line of the Lord's Prayer, "Our Father who are in heaven," or the first line of the 23rd Psalm, "The Lord is my shepherd." Benson's research suggests that persons who use such prayers are much more likely to continue the practice of the relaxation response.

Having become convinced of the special value of using a spiritual intonation as the mantra for the relaxation response, Benson teamed up with Jared Kass, an experienced meditator raised in the Conservative Jewish tradition, to research the value of a spiritual frame of reference for one's psychological health. They constructed a measure of spirituality called the INSPIRIT scale.

Their research found that individuals scoring high in spirituality, as measured by the INSPIRIT scale, received higher scores on tests measuring psychological health. They define spirituality as the feeling that there is *more than just me* and they note that this feeling is not necessarily religious in the traditional sense. Benson believes that his physiological research confirms what religious devotees have maintained all along—prayer has a *special* value! The originators of Eastern meditative practice, the yogin, have maintained for centuries that meditation induces significant perceptual and sensory effects that are preludes to rising consciousness and spiritual integration.

*Alpha Training.* The brain continuously emits electrical microwaves. Hans Berger, a German psychiatrist and researcher, discovered two distinct patterns in these waves. The slower pattern, which consisted of roughly 8 to 10 cycles per second, he called alpha; the faster pattern, 13 to 35 or more cycles per second, he called beta. With equipment sensitive to these tiny waves, researchers have since identified two additional patterns: the theta pattern emits roughly 4 to 7 cycles, and the delta pattern 1 to 3 cycles. Exhibit 3–2 in chapter 3 graphically depicts these waves.

A great deal is now known about the relationship of these patterns to mental activities. Researchers know that beta is associated with worry and active problem-solving; alpha, with relaxation; and theta and delta, with conditions of sleep or coma. Alpha training involves using an electroencephalogram. The alpha waves are developed in visual and auditory forms. Clients are encouraged to do whatever is necessary to cause the electronic light to flash. Although persons differ markedly as to the thoughts they use to produce alpha, the average person learns to produce it in large measure. Since alpha waves signal relaxation, learning to produce them gives the person a powerful tool for relaxing at will.

*Aerobic Exercise.* While aerobic exercise is an effective way of preventing stress buildup, it is also useful in *relieving* stress buildup. Because aerobic exercise was discussed earlier in chapter 3, we will give it but passing attention at this point. Joggers, cyclists, swimmers, and other aerobic exercisers experience the profound relaxation following a period of exercise. The purpose of the stress response is to prepare the person for running or fighting, that is for vigorous action such as aerobic exercise. Stress hormones are effectively dissipated in this manner.

In summary, prescribed breathing, the quieting response, deep muscle relaxation, the relaxation response (and other forms of meditation), alpha training, and aerobic exercise are all promising ways of reducing stress and returning the body to a more relaxed condition. One of these techniques may have more appeal for a given person than the others. Persons should follow their interests in this matter. Experiment with each before settling upon a favorite. All of these methods will result in increased relaxation; all will lead to a less feverish approach to daily activities; all are likely to prove rewarding if they are given a fair trial.

## Putting It All Together

In concluding this chapter we offer a step-by-step program for dealing with serious stressors. This program is primarily designed for highly stressful situations in which constructive action is possible and desirable. The program would look somewhat different if constructed for situations in which no control of the stressor were possible. These steps incorporate many of the suggestions offered throughout the chapter.

Step 1. *Avoid unnecessary changes in your life at this time.* Do not change jobs, get a divorce, take out a mortgage, or make other life changes. Temporarily save your energy for dealing with the stressor. Stabilize your environment and chart a steady course while you are coping with the stressful situation.

Step 2. *Quieten the mind.* Typically, the mind makes things worse at such times by endlessly processing exaggerated versions of the threatening situation. Since the body doesn't know the difference between fact and fantasy, this neurotic thinking heightens arousal. Heightened arousal limits creativity and renders you like a punch drunk boxer who blindly and ineffectively flails away at his opponent.

Bring your thoughts back into the present by centering your attention on your breathing, some sound or visual pattern that invites attention, some repetitive movement, or some prayer. The present is seldom very stressful. What is stressful is the future with its worries about what could happen or the past with its thoughts about what should have happened.

Step 3. *Courageously and aggressively face the stressor.* Don't ignore it. Carefully appraise its seriousness, but don't magnify its threatening properties out of proportion to reality. Avoid such "awfullizing" and "catastrophizing." Ask yourself "What is the worst thing that realistically is likely to happen?" Reassure yourself of all the good things you would still have going for you if the worst thing actually happened; "Well, even if it happened, I'd still have my health, and my job, and my . . . " Try to accept emotionally this worst-case scenario, even though it hasn't actually happened. If you can believe that the most essential elements of yourself and your lifestyle would survive the worst that reasonably could happen, the stressor then will appear far less serious.

Check out the realism of your views of the stressor by consulting with others. Actively seek information from family, friends, and acquaintances. Make a special effort to talk with others who have coped with similar experiences. Overcome any reluctance you may have to let such persons know of your problem, and openly disclose your fears about dealing with it. Listen carefully to their tempering views of the stressor and note any strategies that they have used in successfully coping with it. Too often we fail to obtain information that is critical to coping because we fear that sharing our problems would place us in an unfavorable light.

Step 4. *Take inventory of your coping resources.* Ask yourself "What would I need in order to successfully cope with this situation?" and note how many of the necessary skills and resources you already possess. Spend considerable time thinking about these resources. Be specific. Remind yourself of past successes in dealing with other stressful life situations. Re-live significant aspects of these situations in which you demonstrated the adequacy of your resources. Visualize yourself once again successfully handling the stress. Remind yourself that you managed the stressor quite well although in some of these cases it was not immediately obvious how you were to do it. Give yourself credit for being a good coper. Spend at least half as much time inventorying your resources as you spend considering the stressor. Confidence is a valuable ally in combating stress, and confidence builds on memories of past successes.

Step 5. *Take action!* Commit yourself to some reasonable course of action in dealing with the stressor. Action is itself a powerful stress-reducer, at least initially. Research shows that when facing a stressor the body *lowers* its production of a powerful stress hormone, epinephrine, when the person shifts into action. Therefore, any action taken will lessen the stress initially. Later, however, the value of the action as a stress-reducer will depend on its appropriateness for dealing with the stressor.

Don't avoid taking action out of fear of making the wrong decision. Remind yourself that there are many different ways of successfully dealing with a stressful situation. Also remind yourself that quite often one makes a decision and then makes it the right one by working at it. Obviously, the suggestion to take action is not meant as an endorsement of an impatient, impulsive approach to stressful situations, but rather it is meant to encourage you to take action once you have reasonably researched the problem.

Furthermore, remind yourself that you will never know whether a decision is a correct one until *after* you have made it. You may have a pretty good idea as to its merits, but proof of the "goodness of fit" can only be seen once the consequences of the decision become apparent. Endorse yourself for taking action to reduce or eliminate the stressor. A positive mood energizes us for more effective action against stressors, and self-endorsement contributes significantly to upbeat mood states.

Be open to negative feedback regarding the appropriateness of your action. Even the most studious research of a problem will sometimes lead to inappropriate courses of action. Now and then it will be necessary to recycle and adopt a different course of action.

Step 6. *Take time out to relax.* We have inherited a nervous system that is hypersensitive to potential threat or loss. It is like a wild beast that nervously reacts to everything around it. High states of arousal militate against healthy adjustment. We need to practice methods of taming the nervous system, of returning it to quiescence. At least once or twice each day take time to decompress, to de-escalate through relaxation. There are many effective ways of relaxing. For many, music will work like magic to calm the troubled mind. Some find a quiet walk will do the trick. Others turn to hobbies such as gardening. Yet others use formal methods of relaxing such as prescribed breathing, the quieting response, deep muscle relaxation, the relaxation response, alpha training, prayer, or aerobic exercise.

## Summary

In combating stressors one should first carefully appraise the seriousness of stressors and the adequacy of coping resources, decide whether it is better to coexist with the stressor or try to eliminate it, check one's thinking to refrain from catastrophizing and putting oneself down, and lower wasteful arousal through relaxation procedures. Serious efforts to manage stress will pay rich dividends. Successfully coping leaves us with a greater sense of control over our lives that, in turn, greatly elevates our self-esteem and energizes us for more vibrant living.

## Scoring Key for Correcting Self-talk

1. Reasonable self-statement
2. Self-punishing thinking
3. Blow-up
4. Reasonable self-statement
5. All-or-nothing thinking or self-punishing thinking
6. Reasonable self-statement
7. Reasonable self-statement
8. Personalization
9. Perfectionistic thinking
10. Blow-up
11. Perfectionistic thinking
12. All-or-nothing thinking or self-punishing thinking
13. Projective thinking
14. Selective abstraction
15. Reasonable self-statement

## Interpretive Key for Correcting Self-talk

| No. Correct | Interpretation |
|---|---|
| 12–15 | Brilliant! A modern Sherlock Holmes |
| 9–12 | Outstanding perspicacity. |
| 6–9 | Good work (entitled to one free massage from whomever you can con into doing it). |
| 4–6 | Brush up on your detective work. |
| 3–0 | Let's get with it! |

## ENDNOTES

1. J. Suls and B. S. Fletcher, "Self-Attention, Life, Stress, and Illness: A Prospective Study," *Psychosomatic Medicine* 47 (September/October 1985): 469–481,

2. Adam Smith, *Powers of Mind* (New York: Random House, 1975), 27.

3. Albert Bandura, "Self-Efficacy Mechanism in Human Agency," *American Psychologist* 37, no. 2 (1982): 137–144.

4. Hans Selye, *The Stress of Life* (New York: McGraw-Hill, 1976),

5. Michael Antoni, "Neuroendocrine Influences in Psychoimmunology and Neoplasis: A Review," *Psychology and Health* 1, no.1 (1987): 3–24.

6. Mel Kranzler, *Creative Divorce* (New York: New American Library, 1974).

7. Donald H. Meichenbaum, "A Self-instructional Approach to Stress Manage-

ment: A Proposal for Stress Inoculation Training," in *Stress and Anxiety, vol. 2,* ed. I. Sarason and C. D. Spielberger (New York: Wiley, 1975).

8. Carlos Castenada, *A Separate Reality: Further Considerations with Don Juan* (New York: Pocket Books, 1972).

9. Robert Rosenthal, *Experimenter Effects on Behavior Research* (New York: Appleton-Century-Crofts, 1966).

10. Stanley Schacter and Jerome E. Singer, "Cognitive, Social, and Physiological Determinants of Emotional State," *Psychological Review* 69 (1962): 379–99.

11. Robert Nisbett and Stanley Schacter, "Cognitive Manipulations of Pain," *Journal of Experimental Social Psychology* 2 (1966): 227–36.

12. E. A. Velton, "A Laboratory Task for Induction of Mood States," *Behavior Research and Therapy* 6 (1968): 573–82.

13. D. C. Rimm and S. B. Litvak, "Self-Verbalization and Emotional Arousal," *Journal of Abnormal Psychology* 74 (1969): 181–7.

14. Albert Ellis, "The No Cop-Out Therapy," *Psychology Today* (July 1973): 57.

15. Albert Ellis, "Rational Emotive Therapy and Cognitive Behavior Therapy: Similarities and Differences," *Cognitive Therapy and Research* 4, 326.

16. Aaron T. Beck, *Cognitive Therapy and the Emotional Disorders* (New York: International Universities Press, 1976),

17. S. L. Deal and J. E. Williams, "Cognitive Distortions as Mediators Between Life Stress and Depression in Adolescents. *Adolescence,* 23 (1988): 477–490.

18. Meichenbaum, "Self-instructional."

19. K. Dunlap, *Habits, Their Making and Unmaking* (New York: Liveright, 1932)

20. Victor E. Frankl, "Paradoxical Intention: A Logotherapeutic Technique," *American Journal of Psychotherapy* 14 (1960): 520–535.

21. Martin Ford et al., "Quieting Response Training: Predictors of Long-term Outcome," *Biofeedback and Self-Regulation* 8, no. 3 (1983): 393–408.

22. Robert Levenson, Paul Ekman, and Wallace Friesen, "Voluntary Facial Action Generates Emotion-Specific Autonomic Nervous System Activity," *Psychophysiology* 27, no. 4 (1990): 363–384.

23. Herbert Benson, *The Relaxation Response* (New York: Morrow, 1975).

24. Ibid., 114–115.

25. Herbert Benson, *Beyond the Relaxation Response* (New York: Berkley, 1984).

# PART II

# Strategies for Changing Stressful Lifestyles

# CHAPTER FIVE

# CREATING STRESS-FREE RELATIONSHIPS

"Well, now that we *have* seen each other," said the Unicorn, "if you
believe in me, I'll believe in you. Is that a bargain?"
——Lewis Carroll, *Through the Looking Glass*

Most stress comes from our relationships with others—with spouses,
children, bosses, employees, teachers, students and the like. On the
other hand, a major component of human happiness comes from fulfilling relationships with these same persons. A significant portion of our
time is devoted to achieving and maintaining satisfying relationships.
While most people enjoy time alone, few choose to go for long periods
without seeking the company of others. We are social animals. We
depend upon one another for stimulation, for the performance of
important human functions, and for nourishment. So most of our needs
are met in a social context, and when efforts to meet these needs are
stymied, or even threatened, we respond stressfully. Successful stress
management, then, includes efforts to create nourishing relationships
and to become more skillful in negotiating with others for the meeting
of our needs.

Some people make a mess of their relationships. Their social life
seems made up of one stressful experience after another. Trouble with
the boss, trouble with the spouse or partner, trouble with the children
. . . on and on it goes. Other persons seem to swim in untroubled
waters. They seldom come into conflict with others, and they have

strong social support networks within which their needs are beautifully met. While, admittedly, it is easier to get along with some persons than with others, we authors believe that people largely create the web of relationships that either sustains them or entraps them.

Take persons, for example, who complain of being lonely even when they are with others. Sometimes they create their loneliness by their responses to others. If they lack confidence in their ability to respond intimately, they may actually punish others for making friendly overtures toward them. They abruptly distance themselves from such persons with caustic remarks or gestures. Others then back off as though a friendly paw had been bitten and vow that never again will they run the risk of befriending this person. These lonely persons are usually unaware of having engineered the fractured relationship. They experience relief when the intensity of the relationship no longer requires an intimate response. Even so, they are left once again with their loneliness.

In this chapter we suggest ways of unsnarling tangled relationships and ways of establishing new ones that will be more satisfying both to you and your partners. We highlight the importance of rewarding warmth and thoughtfulness in others, of learning skills useful in negotiating for the meeting of our needs, of helping others to communicate more openly with us, and of learning to express ourselves in ways that reduce confrontation with others.

## One Hand Washes Another

Our needs are more likely to be met if we are attentive to others and reward them for meeting our needs. Persons who realize the rewarding nature of attention and appreciation and use them liberally with others are considered socially alert and impactful. They draw others to themselves like nectar draws bees. Those who fail to use these social rewards, on the other hand, are forced to negotiate for the meeting of their needs without proper currency.

We tend to repeat behaviors which pay off and drop those that do not. This psychological principle probably reflects biological programming for survival. Usually, behaviors that are pleasurable tend to satisfy needs and have survival value. Admittedly, some pleasurable experiences such as the misuse of drugs and overeating are harmful, and some painful experiences such as exercise and surgery are helpful. Generally, though, we are programmed to seek experiences with survival value because they leave us feeling good.

The implication of this principle for getting our needs met is clear. If we want others to meet our needs, then we must reward them for it. If we want others to telephone more often, to visit more often, to write us more often, we must reward them for it. If we want them to allow us greater freedom of movement, we must reward them for it.

The effects of punishment seem short-lived. In the forties, Estes taught rats to trip a lever in order to obtain food pellets.[1] After the habit had been established, he divided the rats into two groups and exposed them to different conditions for extinguishing the habit. One group could continue to trip the lever but this act no longer was rewarded with food. The lever for the second group was wired to produce a slight electrical shock each time it was tripped. As expected, the group that was punished dropped the habit before the nonrewarded group. When, however, both groups were again exposed to the original rewarding condition, the group that had dropped the habit through nonrewarded trials slowly regained the habit, whereas the punished group reestablished the habit *immediately* and *at full strength* when it was discovered that tripping the lever would no longer be punished. Apparently the punished rats had not dropped the habit permanently; they had merely suspended it until assured that they would not longer be punished.

Estes' experiment helps to explain the failure to manage behavior successfully through punishment. Children often resume undesirable habits in spite of frequent efforts to punish them for doing so. Moreover, it is evident that punishment in the form of imprisonment is ineffective in breaking lawless habits as the recidivism rate for released prisoners is somewhere between 65 percent and 80 percent.

We sometimes unwittingly punish others for the very behavior we want from them. Some time ago one of the authors was bike riding with a friend. Suddenly, a small voice yelled out, "Hi, Dad!" He looked around and saw his youngest son waving excitedly to him. The greeting warmed his heart, and he turned and rode back to him. He greeted his son and asked what he was doing. The son replied that he and a friend were skateboarding in the street. At first the author showed interest, but he then proceeded to lecture his son about the dangers of skateboarding in the street. This was enough to kill any enthusiasm the son had earlier shown. After the father resumed the ride, one of his friends chuckled and pointed out how he had effectively punished his son for having warmly greeted him. The feeling of responsibility that parents feel often creates such scenes. Concern comes through as scolding, and children soon may learn to keep their distance.

Unfortunately, the most common way of influencing behavior is through the use of threat. We often ignore the good but notice the bad. Consider the woman who complained to her husband that he was always criticizing her. She asked, "Why don't you ever tell me you like something I've done?" He replied, "You'll know I like it if I don't say anything!" This is standard behavior for some people. They feel awkward with compliments, but are free indeed with criticism.

A few years ago one of the authors participated in a research study in a school system in Appalachia. The researchers were given control of twenty-five classrooms spanning grades one through nine. The goals of the project were to turn negative classrooms into positive ones, to train teachers to lessen their use of aversive control measures, and to increase their use of positive ones. Observations revealed that in addressing students these teachers made thirteen negative references for every positive one. These teachers were caught in the criticism trap. They believed that yelling and screaming at children would get the results they desired, and so they made free use of these aversive controls. In the long run, the more the teachers complained about bad behavior, the more of it they got.

The research team made a concerted effort to encourage teachers to become more positive. After twenty-six weeks of diligent work by the team, the teachers had reversed the ratio. They were now making thirteen positive references for every negative reference. Classroom monitoring showed that the amount of attention the pupils paid in class was directly related to the positiveness of the teacher. At the end of the school year pupils were paying attention 93 percent of the time and had experienced dramatic improvements in their achievement.[2]

## The Pitfalls of Punishment

The chronic use of punishment has unwholesome side effects. For one, it encourages aggressive behavior in others. Animal experimentation has often borne out this fact. Rats placed in cages and randomly shocked first squeal noisily and then scurry about trying to escape. When these maneuvers fail to free them from their painful situation, they then fiercely attack one another.

Perhaps much of the sadism and brutality witnessed in society reflects the chronic punishing conditions to which many public offenders have been subjected. Blatant cases of physical and sexual child abuse readily catch the public's eye, while the chronic negative conditions in which millions of children are reared receive little attention. The twisting and warping of personalities comes not so much from acute traumas but rather from chronic negativism within our homes. In the early years, parents are the most important people in the lives of children. Children look to them for self-validation. If parents subject them to constant criticism and harassment, children interpret this to mean they are not valued and are likely to incorporate such discouraging views into their self-concepts. However well-intentioned the use of chronic punishment may be, its use is likely to destroy the self-esteem of its victims.

Chronic punishment also teaches the victim to escape the punisher. If someone is constantly pointing out our foibles and complaining about our conduct, we may avoid them at all costs. How sad that we may drive loved ones away by our constant negativism. Absenteeism in the class-room, for example, may reflect a student's effort to escape a punishing situation. Thousands of students experience failure daily from classwork that outdistances their academic readiness. Many of these students remain physically in the classroom but escape in their minds.

Many people refrain from using rewards to reinforce good behavior because they believe that this practice constitutes bribery. But rewarding people for good behavior is hardly bribery—it is just good common sense. Parents who believe it is bribery often set up a no-win condition for their children. If children do the wrong thing, they are punished, if they do the right thing, they are ignored. At best they only can break even under this conditioning and learn to avoid risks, to refrain from extending themselves, to play it safe. The resulting personality type is bland, overly cautious, and apathetic.

Although material things such as money and gifts come to mind when we think of rewards, the most powerful rewards often are the attention and appreciation of others. In one study, supervisors were asked to rank morale factors *for their workers*. They ranked them in the following order:

1. Good wages
2. Job security
3. Promotion and growth in the company
4. Good working conditions
5. Work that keeps one interested
6. Personal loyalty to workers
7. Tactful disciplining
8. Full appreciation of work done
9. Sympathetic help on personal problems (respect)
10. Feeling "in" on things

The workers were then asked to rank these morale factors for themselves. The following represents their ranking:

1. Full appreciation of work done
2. Feeling "in" on things
3. Sympathetic help on personal problems (respect)
4. Job security
5. Good wages
6. Work that keeps one interested
7. Promotion and growth in the company
8. Personal loyalty to workers
9. Good working conditions
10. Tactful disciplining

Notice the stark contrast between these two lists. The last three factors on the supervisors' list were elevated to the top of the workers' list. And what do these top three factors have in common? They all related to social rewards—to attention and appreciation. Workers passed up such basics as good wages, job security, and promotion and growth in the company in favor of these social rewards.

People who are skeptical of the importance of social rewards often turn out to be the ones who make least use of them. The force of negative conditioning makes it difficult to notice *good* performance. Becoming a positive person takes time and effort.

# The Power of Appreciation

There are a few rules for the effective use of appreciation. First, it must be genuine. If it does not come from the heart, it likely will be perceived as manipulative. Second, like constructive criticism, it should be directed to a *specific* performance. "I appreciate the fact that you put the dishes in the dishwasher and straightened up the kitchen before you left for work this morning. I know you were in a hurry, and I think it was very considerate of you" is likely to prove more effective than, "You know, Sam, you're a considerate person." There is no specific basis for the last compliment, and, consequently, Sam may brace himself for some request to follow. If appreciation is used loosely and without adequate reason, it will be seen as manipulative and will soon lose its motivating effect.

Third, appreciation should follow *closely* the behavior it is intended to reinforce. Consequences influence behavior more strongly if they are immediate. The longer the interval between the behavior and its consequence, the weaker the effect. This accounts for the persistence of a great deal of self-defeating behavior. Alcoholism is a good example. The immediate consequences of drinking are rewarding. Only later come the hangover, complaints from a spouse, excuses to be made for absence from work, and so on. The medical treatment requires the alcoholic each day to take antabuse, a drug that has an *immediate,* catastrophic effect upon the body when combined with the smallest amount of alcohol. Bringing the punishing consequences closer to the addictive behavior greatly increases its effect.

A reasonable formula for influencing the behavior of others through appreciation includes the following steps:

- Clearly signal what you would like. Express your wishes in terms of preferences rather than demands backed by veiled threats.
- Do not expect perfect compliance with your wishes. Accept approximations of the behavior you want.
- Recognize and reward this accommodating behavior with attention and appreciation.
- Be willing to reciprocate others' behavior with your own accommodations and thoughtfulness.

The skillful use of this formula can significantly improve relationships and make them more likely to be need-satisfying. We are likely to be surprised by our increased effectiveness in influencing the behavior of others.

## Declare Yourself—The Effectiveness of Assertive Behavior

People are often overly tenuous in their responses to each other, even when they have a clear right to be more assertive. The fear of strong responses from others, and the uncertainty over their rights, causes many people to be tentative and fuzzy in their communication. Lack of assertiveness, then, often sets the person up as a patsy to be taken advantage of by less sensitive people.

The worst part about being exploited is the residue of self-contempt with which we are left. We know that we are partly to blame for the exploitation, and we taunt ourselves for our unwillingness to stand up for our rights.

An assertive response is the straightforward, honest expression of what we believe, feel, or want *without* trying to force others to give it to us. This clear signalling is the only viable base for satisfying relations with others. It is difficult to sustain and build relationships based upon exploitation. If we are unable to assert ourselves, to share honestly our feelings with others, we will tend to withdraw from them. If we are unassertive, we make few requests of others for fear that they will make unreasonable requests of us. As a result, many live self-encapsulated lives, defensively insulated against the give and take that characterizes mutually fulfilling relationships.

Many people are uncertain as to how assertive they are. The checklist in Exhibit 5–1 may help. It measures attitudes and responses to (1) one's anger, (2) the anger of others, (3) one's freedom in refusing and making requests, and (4) one's spontaneity in initiating communication with others.[3]

If you do not do too well on the checklist, do not worry. Remember, nobody's perfect. Look over the answers given in the key. On questions where your selections were the same as those given in the key, you probably have no trouble in asserting yourself. Where your answers differ from the key, figure out which of the areas are the most difficult. Then think of specific situations in your life that fit those problem categories. Look at the questionnaire again and try to figure out what irrational beliefs may be blocking your assertiveness.

## Giving Yourself Permission to be Assertive

We must become assertive with ourselves before we can become assertive with others, that is, we must give ourselves permission to become assertive. There are reasons that we fail to be assertive. We may be uncertain about our right to do so, and we may have little confidence in our ability to be assertive in effective, unhurtful ways.

Fuzziness about rights often comes from inappropriately applied cultural training. The culture seems to teach that a selfless kind of humility is virtuous. Such thinking can sometimes be highly nonfunctional. Instead of contributing to respectful, loving relationships, such behavior sometimes inhibits them. When persons surrender their rights, they train others to take advantage of them. Sacrificing rights also results in an overly cautious posture toward others. We do not extend ourselves or take risks with others since we anticipate hurt from them. Manuel Smith in *When I Say No, I Feel Guilty* lists certain personal rights that will

*(Text continued on page 141)*

**Exhibit 5-1.** Assertive Communication Questionnaire

---

*Instructions*: The following questionnaire covers five areas that are often blocks to assertive behavior. There are two questions for each area. The first allows you to assess your attitude and irrational beliefs; the second gives you a chance to examine your behavior. Check one or more answers, as they apply to you.

*Dealing with My Own Anger*
1. When I am angry with people, I usually:
   a. am afraid to say anything directly, because I don't want to hurt their feelings.
   b. am afraid that if I do say something, it will sound aggressive and they won't like me.
   c. feel OK about expressing what is on my mind.
   d. feel anxious and confused about what I want to say.

2. When I am angry with someone, I usually:
   a. drop hints about my feelings, hoping he or she will get the message.
   b. tell the person in a direct way what I want, and feel OK about it.
   c. avoid the person for a while until I calm down and the anger wears off.
   d. blow up and tell him/her off.

*Dealing with Other's Anger*
3. When someone gets angry with me, I usually:
   a. think he/she doesn't like me.
   b. feel too scared to ask why and to try to work things out.
   c. feel confused and want to cry.
   d. think I have a right to understand why he/she is angry and to respond to it.
   e. immediately feel wronged.
   f. feel angry in return.
   g. feel guilty.

4. When someone gets angry with me, I usually:
   a. end up crying.
   b. back off.
   c. ask him/her to explain his/her anger further, or else I respond to it in some other straightforward manner.
   d. get angry in return.
   e. apologize if I don't understand why he/she is angry.
   f. try to smooth it over.
   g. make a joke out of it and try to get him/her to forget the flare-up.

5. When I need time and information from a busy professional, I usually think he or she will:
   a. resent my taking up valuable time.
   b. consider my request as legitimate and be pleased that I'm interested.
   c. act as though he/she doesn't mind but secretly resent me.
   d. make me feel inferior.

---

*(Continued on next page)*

**Exhibit 5–1.** (Continued)

---

6. When I need time and information from a busy professional, I usually:
   a. put off calling until I absolutely have to.
   b. apologize for taking up his/her time when I call.
   c. state directly what I need and ask for what I want.
   c. let him/her know that I expect immediate attention. After all, I'm important too.

*Refusing Requests*
7. If someone asks me to do a favor for him/her and I refuse, I think he/she probably will:
   a. hate me.
   b. be angry with me.
   c. understand and will not mind.
   d. act as though he/she doesn't mind, but secretly resent me.
   e. think I don't like him/her.
   f. hesitate to ask me again.

8. If someone asks me to do them a favor and I don't want to do it, I usually:
   a. do it anyway.
   b. let him/her know that I resent the request, but do it grudgingly.
   c. tell him/her I'd rather not do it.
   d. tell him/her I'd rather not do it, and apologize profusely.

*Making Requests*
9. When I need something from someone else, I usually feel:
   a. as though I shouldn't bother her/him by asking.
   b. as though people don't really want to do things for me.
   c. as though I don't want to put him/her on the spot by asking.
   d. that it's OK to go ahead and ask.
   e. afraid to ask, because he/she might say no.
   f. as though he/she should do what I want.

10. When I need something from someone else, I usually:
    a. don't ask unless I'm absolutely desperate.
    b. ask and apologetically explain why I need help.
    c. do nice things for him/her, hoping the favor will be returned.
    d. become demanding and insist on getting my way.
    e. ask directly for what I want, knowing that he/she can refuse my request if he/she wants to.

*Initiating Communication*
11. When I walk into a party where I don't know anyone, I usually think:
    a. that no one there will talk to me.
    b. that everyone else is relaxed except me.
    c. that I'm out of place, and everyone knows it.l
    d. that I won't be able to say the right thing if someone does talk to me.
    e. of ways to get attention.

---

*(Continued on next page)*

**Exhibit 5-1.** (Continued)

---

12. When I walk into a party where I don't know anyone, I usually:
    a. wait for someone to come and talk to me.
    b. introduce myself to someone who looks interesting.
    c. stay on the sidelines and keep to myself.
    d. put a lamp shade on my head or otherwise behave in a bizarre manner, hoping someone will notice.
    e. rush for food or drink or a cigarette to make it look as if I'm busy and having a good time.

---

*Source:* From L. Z. Bloom, K. L. Coburn, and F. C. Pearlman, *The New Assertive Woman* (New York: Delacorte, 1975), by permission.

---

## KEY FOR SCORING QUESTIONNAIRE

The following answers on the questionnaire indicate assertive beliefs and behaviors:

| | |
|---|---|
| 1. c | 7. c |
| 2. b | 8. d |
| 3. d | 9. d |
| 4. c | 10. e |
| 5. b | 11. e |
| 6. c | 12. b |

---

*(Text continued from page 138)*
help to thwart the manipulation of others. Among these are the following:

- The right to change your mind.
- The right to make mistakes.
- The right to say "I don't know" or "I don't understand".
- The right to decide whether or not to help others with their problems.
- The right to offer no excuses or justifications for your behavior.
- The right to judge your own behavior, thoughts, and emotions and to take responsibility for them.[4]

We would add that we have the right to make requests of others. This does not mean that we can or will always get our own way. Still, there is nothing wrong or pushy about expressing preferences. Indeed, it is better than suppressing them and sulking as a result. There is little chance that others will meet our needs if they do not know that we have them. Quite often, we are afraid to express wants for fear of rejection. Consequently, we withhold wants and then fault others for not meeting them. This attitude is obviously doomed to failure.

We also have the right to refuse the request of others. There is no virtue in saying "Yes" if we cannot say "No." In the long run we will prove more interesting to others and our relationships will be more rewarding if we exercise both the option to say "Yes" *and* the option to say "No." No one respects a pushover. When we do choose to accommodate an unpleasant request of another, we might sensitively point out that we are not fond of doing so but are responding out of love or respect for the other person. This will make others less likely to take advantage of us and more likely to respond favorably to future requests from us.

## Viewing the Costs of Being Assertive Objectively

A second hurdle to self-assertion is the presumed cost of doing so. Most nonassertive persons greatly overestimate the costs of responding assertively to others. They may believe that standing up for their own rights, honestly expressing opinions and preferences, or saying "no" to others will cost them a friendship, a marriage, or a job. While the costs are sometimes real, our views of them are usually disproportionate to reality. Moreover, persons may fear their own reaction to the rebuttal of others. They may imagine the rebuttal to be far stronger than their assertion. Because others may see them as "acting out of character," their early attempts at assertion may elicit strong responses from others. Their greatest fear may be that they will fall apart under the heat of the exchange and appear weak and irrational to others. Once again, such unfortunate scenarios are possible but not necessarily likely. One can guard against this likelihood by first practicing assertive responding in relatively nonthreatening situations. The idea is to try out the skills first with less-threatening persons and in less-threatening situations before walking into the lion's cage. Remember, although we have a right to express ourselves, we obviously do not have a right to have our way *all* the time.

When faced with an array of possible responses, we should choose the *least intense* response that will get the job done. Threatening another person into compliance is done at the expense of making an enemy. The goal in all interpersonal situations is harmonious relationships, which are characterized by fairness. Unnecessarily strong expressions are foolishly wasteful of precious human energy.

Self-assertions should be viewed in the context of friendship skills. In order to maintain friendships, we must sometimes acquiesce to the requests of others, even when we would prefer not to. Assertiveness is not meant to be an excuse for selfishness. Living in society requires consideration of others.

People who feel powerless and exploited often experience more conflict than people who feel secure and strong. If we are confident of our ability to take care of ourselves, we often give off signals that discourage others from manipulative actions. Moreover, if we feel strong, we do not need to engineer arguments in order to develop the skills of self-defense. Nonassertive persons appear overly sensitive to potential exploitation. More secure people do not attend to minor clues of potential exploitation because they have confidence in their ability to take care of themselves. When insecure people encourage conflict, they are often seen as masochistic or desirous of inflicting pain on themselves. These people seem to pick fights and then lack the skills to defend themselves. While they seem to be seeking punishment, they are more likely to be seeking opportunities to learn to defend themselves. Unfortunately, their lack of skill condemns them to additional losing experiences and further confirms their feelings of inadequacy and weakness.

Assertiveness includes the ability to express affection as well as irritation. Some people need more help in expressing warmth and affection than in expressing anger. They appear awkward and embarrassed with the direct expression of affection. Consequently, they avoid such direct expressions in favor of indirect expressions that are often missed by others. Since many people hold unhandsome self-images, they are quite sensitive to disapproval but insensitive to expressions of warmth. They miss subtle expressions of affection because they are not set up emotionally to receive them. Therefore, it is often necessary to make expressions of warmth, affection, and love quite explicit. Otherwise, people may live with others for years without being certain that they are cared for deeply.

## Learning the Techniques of Being Assertive

Once we accept the idea that we have some rights, too, then we must decide on the most effective ways of asserting. The manner of asserting depends on the kind of relationship sought with the other person. There are basically three types of relationships in which assertive responses become appropriate: (1) long-range relationships, where it is important to maintain consideration and respect; (2) short-range exploitative relationships that are totally unimportant; and (3) relationships wherein the other person, for whom we have no deep caring, is constantly critical. Furthermore, each of these situations calls for a different kind of assertive response.

## Kelley-Winship Model

Jan Kelley and Barbara Winship have proposed a three-part assertive response that is most appropriate for situations in which we are seeking to find and maintain a high degree of caring and respect[5]. According to this model, the assertive response should include an empathy component, a conflict component, and an action component. The empathic part of the response is recognition of what the other person is feeling. The conflict part is a statement of what we are feeling. And the action part is what we want to happen. The following example highlights these components. "Jane, I know you're working some overtime at the office these days, and I realize that it would be convenient if I'd pick up your share of the chores around here (empathy). But the way I look at it is that I'm paying my share of the rent and doing my share of the chores (conflict), so I don't plan to do your work, too (action).

In such situations we have the right to be far more direct if we choose. We could, of course, merely say, "You do your own damn chores!" We have the right, but we would undoubtedly have to pay for such insensitive bluntness with injury to the relationship. The three-part response softens the statement without obliterating its clarity.

It is important to let the other person know that his or her position is understood. People sometimes persist in their requests because they assume that the other person is not hearing or understanding them. They are more apt to accept refusal gracefully if they know the other person has gotten the message, if the other person acknowledges its importance. Acknowledging the basis of another's request through the empathic component tends to take the drive out of a persistent request, and it also signals respect in that we have bothered to listen and understand.

It is also respectful of us to share the basis for our decisions regarding the requests of others. This often makes it easier for others to accept the decision. The following illustration helps to underline the importance of the conflict component. A dorm mate bounces into a fellow student's room and tries to persuade him to have a couple beers with him at the local bar. Wanting to preserve the friendship, the student replies, "John, I know you're feeling good and just want to be friendly (empathy), but you see, I've got this test in the morning, and I'm really worried about it (conflict), so I want to study quietly for the next couple of hours. Perhaps we could celebrate with a couple beers after that (action)?" Letting the other person know the reason for turning down a request is likely to appear less arbitrary and, consequently, less rejecting.

It is equally important to include an unequivocal action component. If we stop with the conflict component, we merely invite the other person to try to outflank our logic. When this happens, the likelihood of counterarguments increases the chance of ego damage to one or the other of us. It is much better to conclude with a solid action statement. Do not finish the action component with a lilt in the voice. This indicates indecisiveness, and, again, it invites argument.

## Broken Record

Smith suggests the Broken Record technique for situations where we are being exploited by sales representatives, service managers, and the like.[6] The technique involves stating over and over again what it is we want. Calmly repeat, "But the merchandise is faulty, and I want a refund" or "I know you tried, but I want you to adjust the timing so that the engine doesn't ping." The technique, when mastered, allows us, while sticking to the desired point, to feel comfortable in ignoring manipulative verbal side traps, argumentative baiting, and irrelevant logic. In this way we can persist at a point without having to rehearse arguments or suffer angry feelings beforehand in order to be up for an assertive scene.

Sometimes an exploiter is equipped with two or three counterarguments, which can cause an unprepared person to fold. The situation can be turned around, however, by performing like a broken record. Merely restate the demand repeatedly in a calm manner, which usually causes the exploiter to acquiesce after having spent the sum of the arguments he is prepared to offer. Such scenes involve contests of wills, and the person best prepared mentally to persevere often wins. If the technique is used appropriately, the script may look something like this:

*You:* "Hi, I purchased this shirt here last week. When I tried it on, I discovered it was defective. I'm returning it, and I would like a refund."

*Clerk*: "I'm sorry, sir, but we can't accept returned merchandise without a sales slip."

*You*: "No problem, I've got the sales slip right here."

*Clerk*: "Well, what seems to be wrong with the shirt? It's one of the very best we carry, and we just never have anyone unhappy with this brand."

*You*: "The lapel is creased improperly. Since it is permanent press, there is little chance that I could successfully correct the crease by ironing it—so I'd just like to get a refund."

*Clerk*: "Well, the crease doesn't look improper to me. It's hard to get them to match up perfectly. In fact, it looks pretty good to me. I'm sure no one will notice it."

*You*: "Yeah, well, it looks funny to me, and I'm the one who has to wear it. So I want a refund."

*Clerk*: "Well, it's awfully inconvenient, this sort of thing. We'll have to get the manager's approval, and you might have to wait around awhile."

*You*: "Well, I want the refund, so you had better see the manager."

Notice that it was necessary to persistently repeat the request over each of the clerk's objections. You merely outlasted him. This is important in such situations. We should prepare ourselves beforehand by giving ourselves permission to make the request. We should remind ourselves that we have a perfect right to make the request. Moreover, we should expect some objections from the clerk and be prepared to make a request like a broken record.

## Fogging

Many people suffer enormously from the chronic criticism of others. Such people lack the assertive skills to cope comfortably with nagging. Consequently, they recoil defensively from the onslaught and often change their behavior to satisfy the demands. The result is often bitter disappointment. They fault themselves for their cowardice, but seem helpless in the face of such criticism.

Smith recommends fogging as a technique for handling criticism.[7] We accept the criticism by calmly admitting the possibility or probability of some truth in it without indicating any need to change the behavior. The technique allows us to receive criticism comfortably without becoming anxious or defensive and without rewarding the person who criticizes. Criticism is usually manipulative. The critic is seeking a behavioral change. If we accept the possibility of the accuracy of the criticism without indicating a disposition to change the offending behavior, the critic wins an empty victory.

Through fogging we remain the judge of what we will do and destroy the automatic connection between the criticism and any change in behavior that is anticipated by the critic. The critic believes, as a result of past experience, that we will automatically change if we recognize the validity of the criticism. The critic is taken back, bewildered by our lack of any need to change the behavior in order to erase the criticism. Often the critic will repeat the charge as though we did not understand what was said. Eventually the critic learns that the victory is not worth the battle, that we cannot be manipulated by this cleverly directed criticism. The following is an example of fogging:

*Critic*: "You're late! You're a half hour late? I've stood around here waiting for you while I could have been inside bowling a warm-up line with the team."

*You*: "You're right. I'm a good half hour late. I told you I didn't want to practice before the match. Why didn't you just go on in and join the others?"

*Critic*: "Damn it, you were late last week, too."

*You*: "I believe I got here fifteen or twenty minutes late last week. You're right again."

*Critic*: "Well, I'm not waiting for any half hour next week. You can bet on that."

*You*: "Good, that's smart. You go on in and warm-up with the team, and I'll get here as early as I conveniently can. As always, I'll be here before the match begins."

*Critic*: "Well, I want you to come early so we can go in together. I don't like going in without you."

*You*: "I like being with you, too, Charlie, but I'm not going to break my neck to get here that early. I'm not asking you to adjust to my schedule, so you just go on in, and I'll be along pretty soon."

It is clear that Charlie wanted something more than a confession of tardiness. He wanted a schedule-change that would conform to his. The critic assumes that he can get his way only if he can verbally outmaneuver others. He attacks their behavior through his "logical" criticism, and he fully expects others to cave in to his demands when his position proves superior to theirs. Fogging is a way of destroying this automatic connection between acknowledged criticism and behavior change. Destroying this connection leaves the critic nonplussed and, perhaps, angrily respectful of our control over our own behavior.

Fogging is not necessarily the preferred way of handling criticism. Often we want to be more responsive to criticism if we seek to build friendships. Living is a matter of getting and giving, which means that we sometimes accommodate the reasonable requests of friends and loved ones. Still, there are times when we must establish sovereignty over our own behavior. This can be done by making the point that we alone are responsible for what we choose to do, that we cannot be coerced into disagreeable courses of action by manipulative criticism. And when this is the point that needs to be made, fogging is the preferred response to criticism.

## Nonverbal Assertiveness

Our appearances often contradict our statements. In order to make a message effective, we must match nonverbal expressions with verbal ones. Fear often causes us to mute the impact of strong statements with a smile, a lilt in the voice, or a placating posture. More often than not, we are unconscious of these conflicting signals. We sense that words are strong medicine and fear the consequences. Often we fear the guilt that our conscience may inflict for speaking strongly to someone else, and we fear the other person's reaction. When we are uncertain of being able to cope with these consequences, we unconsciously destroy the impact with contradictory nonverbal signals.

It is easy to see the weakening influence of these nonverbal signals. Remember seeing someone smile while telling another that his behavior is offensive? What was the effect of the smile on the verbal message? Did the smile weaken the message? The smile allows the other person to conclude that we are not very serious in the expression of irritation. The smile is likely to be taken more seriously than our words. The other person may think that we are merely joking, or that we are unsure of our point, or that our protest is but a good-natured jab that has no real significance.

But if our irritation is serious enough to be expressed, then the words and the nonverbal signals should be unequivocal. Check your facial expression in the mirror while practicing an assertive response. If only the facial signals were read, what would they be saying? Later it will not be necessary to check in this mechanical manner, but it may prove helpful for a while.

Eye messages are also important communication signals. Poor eye contact is likely to destroy an assertive verbal response. To measure the effect of failing eye contact, have a friend role-play the following script in two ways. First, have the friend look furtively while repeating the line, "You cut in front of me, and I want you to go to the end of the line." Now have the friend repeat the same words with solid eye contact. Which of the two performances is likely to have the greatest effect? Poor eye contact is generally interpreted as being indicative of fearfulness and lack of self-confidence. If you give yourself poor marks for your eye contact, you can significantly improve your assertiveness by practicing before a mirror. Be careful not to appear to stare in a hostile way at the other person. Proper eye contact is merely meant to connote straightforward, honest communication, not hostility.

Body posture is also a form of communication. Crossed arms and legs suggest defensiveness and resistance. Leaning backward away from the other suggests fearfulness or resistance. Slouching suggests casualness and lack of intensity.

The quality of the voice is one of the more important aspects of communication; it is very sensitive to fear. Fear often affects the natural rhythm, pitch, and intensity of the voice. When fearful, the voice may stammer, speed up into a rapid-fire, machine-gun style, or slow down. The pitch usually rises in shrillness, but sometimes it lowers to a whisper. Furthermore, the voice may become very loud. While no one of these voice changes is incontrovertible proof of fearfulness, the combination of two or more of them most often signals fear. To properly diagnose the effects of vocal qualities upon an intended message, tape the voice in simulated assertive situations and listen for its impact.

## Openly Communicating With Others

Often, the essence of our message to others gets lost in the overtones of the language we use. We think we have clearly signalled our intentions or feelings. However, communication involves both *sending* and *receiving* the message. It is quite possible for the content of a message to be entirely missed by the other person as a result of the defensiveness triggered in him or her by the language and style of expression of a message.

Sometimes we have trouble *receiving* a message. The problem may lie either within ourselves or within another. The more threatened people are, the fuzzier and more imprecise they are in expressing themselves. People may be afraid to be understood. They may remain fuzzy for fear their opinions will not be well received if they are clearly understood. They fear that others may ridicule them or become angry if they express themselves clearly, so they keep all options open by speaking in vague generalities.

It is in the interest of clearer communication for us to work at reducing the threat that others experience in expressing themselves. It helps greatly if we are able to assume an open, nonjudgmental stance while listening. It is not necessary to embrace the opinions of the other person; it is enough that we try to understand them.

It is also possible that trouble in understanding other people may lie within ourselves. We may be resisting the weight of another's position because we sense that the logic of our own position may suffer. We may conclude that another's opinions do not make sense, when in reality, they may make so much sense that they undermine our own opinions. The antidote to this resistance is a willingness to readjust our opinions in the face of new or conflicting information. A person unwilling to change may persistently resist counterarguments by feigning misunderstanding.

## Respectfully Attending to Others

There are certain behaviors that facilitate the open communication of others. We can respectfully attend to others when they are expressing themselves; we can respond in a way that lets them know they are understood; and we can show further interest by initiating considerations that they may not have entertained.

*Attending* is a matter of positioning ourselves so that we reward the other person for self-disclosure. It involves listening to the full message being expressed. Most people feel that someone is paying attention only when that person is squarely facing them, shows good eye contact, and assumes a receptive posture. Check this out when talking to someone. Have the person position his or her body at an oblique angle from you while you are talking about a personal matter. Notice that it is more satisfying if the other person turns around to face you squarely.

Now have the other person avoid eye contact by focusing on the floor or ceiling. Notice how difficult it is for you to continue your story. Now ask someone to cross both legs and arms while you are talking. Does the person appear resistant in this posture? While such posturing may seem too elementary to be significant, it is just such basics that give others cues for judging whether or not the listener is interested in their expression of opinion. Moreover, it is often helpful if the listener suspends potentially distractive behaviors such as smoking, gum chewing, and finger twiddling. Eliminating these behaviors frees us to concentrate more on the message and causes the speaker to feel more fully attended to than otherwise.

Attending is also a matter of reading the other person's nonverbal signals. Look the other person over. What is the energy level? Is the person down? How far down? Is there anxiety? Fidgeting? Quivering? Ask yourself, "How am I when I look that way?" With practice we can learn to trust ourselves in deciphering nonverbal signals.

Attending also involves listening to a spoken message. We must listen for both content and feeling. Most people are better at ferreting out content than feeling. To understand a feeling properly, we must combine the spoken content with the nonverbal signals. Listen for the central themes. Try to understand the circumstances surrounding the feelings expressed. Silently rehearse what has been said and then ask, "What would be important to me about this message if I had said it?" Learn to listen empathically for the other person's perceptions of things. It is as though we crawl inside the other person's skin and look at the world as he or she sees it. By so doing, the truly important aspects of the situation begin to emerge in clearer outline.

## Responding That Releases Stifled Expression

We can further reward others for their openness by responding to their disclosure in a way that lets them know that they are understood. It is not enough merely to understand; we must convey this understanding through accurate responding. In the same way that we attend to content and feeling in a message, we must acknowledge both in our response. If we can accurately combine the essence of the feeling and the content in a short response, we encourage the person to continue his or her story. A simple way of doing this is to make various adaptations of what the person has said, possibly in the following format: "You feel _____ because _____." Where a feeling can be expressed in a single adjective, be sure to use feeling words rather than thinking words. The sentence, "You feel that you are not going to be able to make it," is a description of thinking, not feeling. If this is what a person is thinking, he or she might be feeling discouragement, depression, or despair. Discouragement, depression, and despair are feeling words. Since people want others to understand what they are feeling, responding with a feeling word is particularly rewarding. Often these succinct responses will clarify matters considerably for others and encourage them to delve further into the matter.

However simple this approach may seem, one thing is certain—it is not practiced often, widely, or well. Let us assume that a close friend says, "I don't know whether I want to try to discuss it with you again. It never seems to help. I honestly think it makes matters worse. We no more than get started until we're shouting at one another. Somehow or other what we start talking about gets lost in the process, and we just end up angry at one another. I know it's important, and I really wish we could work through it. But trying just seems to make things worse. And yet, I don't think I can go on indefinitely this way." If our purpose is to demonstrate an understanding of the feeling and content of this disclosure and to encourage the person to continue this story in an open, honest manner, which of the following responses is likely to be most effective?

*Response 1*:  "Well, it's obvious that you've given up. You've just written me off, and you don't really care what happens to our friendship."

*Response 2*:  "You seem really worried because we can't seem to resolve issues like this. Nothing we do appears to you to help much, and arguing like this is really punishing."

Response 2 is much more likely to encourage someone to keep talking, to try to work it out, than is Response 1. Response 1 shows a great deal of hurt and defensiveness and would likely rekindle the heat of the argument or increase the extent of a friend's despair. Response 2, on the other hand, indicates that we have listened well, that we sense a friend's discouragement and bewilderment. It admits to a realization that the friend has not written us off, that his or her discouragement is mentioned only to solicit our efforts to unravel this gordian knot. Respect and caring are indicated by this nondefensive response. While nothing is ultimately predictable in human relations, this second response seems more likely to encourage the other person to continue.

Facilitative responses often include both the feeling and content of a person's statement. While either the feeling or the content can sometimes be adequate, a fuller response that includes both is often superior. Consider another example: Suppose you have had a very difficult time at the office and are licking your wounds and seeking a nourishing response from your spouse. You say, "I don't know why I was stupid enough to allow them to talk me into taking the manager's job. I sometimes wonder if I'm cut out to take all the gaff. I'll bet I had ten customer complaints, and every damn one of them was a lulu." You pause, and your spouse replies:

*Response 1*: "Well, you didn't have to accept the job, you know. I never asked you to take it. I've never complained about the money we've had to live on."

*Response 2*: "Sounds like you've had a bad day and you want a little sympathy."

*Response 3*: "Ten! Boy, that's a lot more complaints than you usually get, isn't it?"

*Response 4*: "If you don't like the job, why don't you just quit? With your skills you can always get another one."

*Response 5*: "You feel tired and worried that maybe this job is going to be more of a hassle than you bargained for."

Which of these responses is most likely to encourage further examination of the situation? While the first response might cause anger, the second would likely cause embarrassment and a slight sense of belittlement. The third seems somewhat irrelevant. The fourth is supportive and may at some point be productive, but it also may be too radical for the moment. The fifth response is the most likely to be facilitative. It identifies both the feelings and content of the disclosure. It does not attempt to solve the problem. It merely indicates that the spouse has listened and deeply understood what was said. Frankly, it is not often that we receive such facilitative responses from others. People often must move ahead with their stories over the disinterested, oblique, and irrelevant responses of others. Such responses leave us feeling alone and isolated, and we persist only under the most dire of circumstances.

Sometimes we can help further by initiating considerations that the other person may not have yet considered. Timing is of utmost importance in determining whether such initiation will prove helpful or hurtful. When solutions are suggested or contradictory aspects of a disclosure or admonishments are given before a great deal of attending and responding is done, the timing is premature, and the outcome is likely to be unfortunate.

The establishment of a warm and caring relationship is absolutely basic to being able to initiate suggestions. This kind of a relationship can be stretched without breaking because it has a certain elastic quality to it. Still, if we do not attend and respond sufficiently, the initiation of additional considerations may strain the relationship beyond its ability to remain intact.

## Adult Communication

People often find themselves involved in confrontations that they do not understand at all. There is a certain inevitability about the outcomes of some efforts to communicate with others. It is as though the communication is scripted or programmed to turn out in some hurtful way. Worse yet, we sense the way something is going to turn out from the beginning of the discussion. We sense what is going to happen; it seems inevitable; and yet, we play the script again and again.

There is much insight to be gained from Transactional Analysis about such impasses. Transactional analysis (TA) is a psychotherapeutic system for analyzing communication. Its founder Eric Berne applied his understanding of Freudian and Adlerian psychology to communication analysis.[8] The system is elegant in its simplicity and relevance. It assumes that people communicate from one of three attitudinal postures, which are called ego states. These ego states—*parent, adult,* and *child*—elicit differing responses in others. These ego states, or postures, are to be found in each of us, and within the course of a single day, we may shift into each of them many times.

The meaning of these three ego states is quite easily understood since the roles called for are common to our experiencing. The parent is that part of the personality that represents the attitudes that we perceived in our parents. The do's and don'ts that they demanded of us as a child are now a part of our conscience. The parent has two faces: the nourishing parent and the critical parent. Most people have been fortunate enough to have had parents who were, to some extent, nourishing. They cared, they watched over their children protectively, and they wanted the best for them. Normally we internalize this same nourishing attitude and pass it on to others. But parents are critical as well as nourishing. In the role of the critical parent, they preach, exhort, and scold.

The adult is that aspect of our functioning that is concerned with solving problems or completing tasks. It is highly objective. It asks who, what, when, where, and why. It does not point fingers, nor does it preach sermons. It is reality-oriented and, consequently, is the best posture to assume when trying to negotiate with others.

The child, like the parent, has two faces. As the natural child, we respond openly, spontaneously, and honestly to others. We are often affectionate and vivacious. As the adaptive child, we often show the puckish, selfish, rebellious or withdrawing side of our nature.

We can analyze communication difficulties by identifying the parent, adult, or child postures we assume while talking with others. Things generally go smoothly as long as we assume the posture the other person is anticipating. Transactions that conform to anticipated postures are called *uncrossed transactions* and look like this:

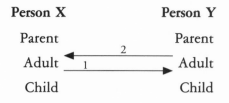

Transactions that do not conform to expected postures are called *crossed transactions* and look like this:

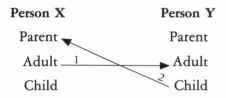

Crossed transactions often cause trouble; they cause us to become defensive. To illustrate this, let us assume that a husband pulls into his driveway about 5 p.m. and begins to make preparations to change the oil in his car. He suddenly realizes that his wife may have supper ready, in which case it will soon be necessary to scrub before eating. Consequently, it would not be wise to begin changing the oil. He cracks open the kitchen door and yells, "June, is supper about ready?" Assuming he has no ulterior reason for asking, his transactional posture is that of the adult, and he is directing his question to another adult posture. Let us assume that the abruptness of the question, coupled with the emotional residue of earlier arguments with the children, causes the wife to feel hassled by the question. Perhaps at this point, she responds, "Will you please leave me alone? Just get off my back! You're always pressuring me to do this or that. I'm doing the best I can." To this point the transaction now looks like this:

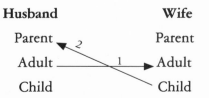

This transaction is crossed. The husband had meant to come from his adult to his wife's adult, but she came from her child to what she hopes will be his nourishing parent. Since he is likely to be angered by this child response when he expected an adult one, her response may indeed hook his parent—but it is likely to be a *critical* parent rather than a nourishing parent. Now let us assume that the husband responds critically by saying, "Well, it's because you never seem to take the initiative and do things on your own. And why the hell are you so touchy anyway?" Now the transactions look like this:

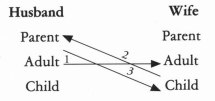

At this point an argument may begin. Both may levy charges against one another, and in the end, both may come out losers.

But let us suppose this situation turned out differently. Aside from the obvious insensitivity of the first ill-timed question, the husband erred yet a second time when he allowed his parent to be hooked. Let us go back to his wife's response of "Will you please leave me alone? Just get off my back! You're always pressuring me to do this or that. I'm doing the best I can." Suppose that the husband senses the hurt she is feeling and remains calm. He remains in the adult and refuses to allow his critical parent to be hooked. He comes back with, "Gee, honey, I'm sorry. I didn't mean to hassle you. I was about to change the oil in the car, and I thought I'd better check with you to see if supper was about ready before I got my hands dirty. I guess it did seem quite abrupt, my poking my head in the door and questioning you right off." The likelihood that this honest, straightforward adult remark will be rewarded is reasonably good. She may catch herself on the heels of his last response and say, "I'm sorry, too, honey, but you wouldn't believe the day I've had!" Now the transactions look like this:

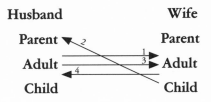

There is now opportunity for the husband to shift back and forth between his adult and nourishing parent, and, if all goes well, the wife will feel attended to, and the husband will get his supper after all.

There are two things that become clear from this illustration: (1) people have more control over their relations with others than they sometimes believe, and (2) staying in the adult often keeps us out of trouble. Each person plays a significant role in influencing how others are going to respond. Still, this statement must be qualified: people are not puppeteers who mechanically pull the strings of puppets. They *influence* — not *determine* — the responses of others. As in the hypothetical illustration, the reaction of others is often influenced by factors over which we have no control. When we engage another, we may still be dealing with unresolved anger from situations in which we perceive that we were belittled. Remarks made in such cases may be the precipitating occasion for venting pent-up hostility. We become the target for delayed shots that should have been directed at others. Even in such cases, however, we are apt to make the situation better or worse, depending upon our communication postures. Suppose Sarah has packed in her anger all day long because she has been afraid to direct it toward her supervisor at work for fear of being fired. Now, suppose she is just looking for battle on the home turf. After a series of increasingly hostile remarks, she says "Damn it, seems like everything around here is left for me to do!" While it is difficult in such situations to predict with accuracy the effect of any response, would you agree that the response triggered by the two following replies are likely to be different?

*First Reply*:    "I swear, all you ever do is complain. You're always complaining about something. It doesn't make any difference what it is. If it's not repairing something around the house, then it's likely to be the finances or the children."

*Second Reply*:    "Honey, you seem really upset about something, and I don't think it's just the work around the house. You seem to be dealing with something else that's bothering you. Maybe you'd like to tell me about it?"

While the second reply may merely trigger further anger on the part of the spouse, it is at least headed in the right direction. It comes from the adult. It contains no venom, no sermons, and it acknowledges the facts. At least it allows for the possibility that Sarah will back off from the "sham" fight and begin to deal with the underlying cause—her anger with the supervisor.

Perhaps another illustration will help. Let us suppose that we are trying to help a friend who is angry with his boss. He says, "I feel like clobbering him." Which of the following responses would seem most helpful?

*Parent*: "John, why don't you grow up. You know you'll be looking for a new job if you punch the boss."

*Adult*: "I can see you're really angry with the boss. Why don't you tell me more about it?"

*Child*: "I wish you would clobber him. There's not a supervisor in the whole damn corporation that I would like to see stomped as much as old Smith."

Most therapists would feel that the only viable response in such situations is the adult one. The parent response is likely to be seen for what it clearly is—belittlement. The child response may encourage a friend to take precipitous action and get himself in serious trouble. Even if he does not follow up on the childish response, he is likely to think the person who offers it is even more impulsive and irresponsible than he is. He may enjoy the support of the childish response, but he will sense danger in talking with someone who responds in this irresponsible manner when he is so upset. The adult response gives him license to further express his emotions, to document the basis for his anger. Most persons think more rationally and deal more realistically with their problems when they have had an opportunity to talk freely about them.

Analyzing our responses to others helps in creating more satisfying relations with them. We can get help in analyzing our responses by constructing an Egogram. An Egogram is a subjective analysis of the percentage of time we respond to others from each of the transactional postures. We should ask ourselves, "How much of the time do I speak from each of these postures?":

| %_____ | %_____ | %_____ | %_____ | %_____ |
|---|---|---|---|---|
| Critical Parent | Nourishing Parent | Adult | Natural Child | Adaptive Child |

If we come at others from our critical parent most of the time, we are likely to place them on the defensive. They are going to feel the one-up-manship and be irritated by it. They may not uncover the basis for their irritation, but they will relate to us based on the response. If, on the other hand, we assume the role of the whining, dependent, adaptive child most of the time, we set others up to care for us, and, at the same time, to more solidly place us in the child's role. Therefore, relations with others are likely to be more satisfying if the higher percentages on the Egogram hover around the center of the axis—that is around the adult, the nourishing parent, and the natural child.

Some insight can be gained into problems with a spouse or friends if an Egogram is constructed for them also. As an example, if a spouse comes from his or her critical parent much of the time, while you are attempting to communicate from an adult posture, a great deal of difficulty can be expected. Both of you are likely to be unhappy with each other. You are likely to be unhappy with the constant complaining and pessimism of your spouse, and your spouse may be disappointed with your seeming blandness or lack of color.

## Self-expression That Reduces Stressful Confrontation

Some semanticists, scientists who study the meaning of words, suggest that people trigger confrontation with others by the use of words that seem to make statements about reality rather than express opinions. This way of speaking makes heavy use of forms of the verb "to be." To avoid this communication bombshell, they recommend we use English Prime, that is English without forms of the verb "to be."

Forms of the verb "to be," such as "is," "are," "was," "were," "will be," or "shall be," all imply reality, not opinion. People can argue about the nature of "reality," but they cannot argue about the expression of an opinion. We can express our opinion about the wisdom of another's opinion, but we cannot tell another that it is **not** his or her opinion. Consider, for example the differences between the following set of expressions:

*First Expression*:     "Bergman's movie, *Face to Face,* is another example of the worthless, pseudophilosophical trash that he has directed over the past twenty years."

*Second Expression*:     "I didn't enjoy Bergman's movie, *Face to Face.* In fact, I haven't enjoyed a single movie he has produced over the past twenty years."

Can you see the difference between the two expressions? In the first statement, the person is presuming to judge the merits of the film, to tell others how it *really* is. This kind of arrogance invites others to argue about Bergman's virtuosity as a director. If they happen to like Bergman, they may pick up the gauntlet and do battle. In the second expression, however, the person presumes to be an expert about one thing only—his or her opinion. Since we cannot know for certain what another person feels or believes, there is really no room to argue about the matter. It is ridiculous to counter with, "No, you don't believe that! You actually enjoy his works." Now consider another example.

*First Expression:*     "You are very inconsiderate. Let's face it, John, you never once consider my wishes in such matters. You brush aside my wants and do precisely what you want."

*Second Expression*:  "You know, John, I feel hurt when I think my wants are being ignored. It seems to me that you brush aside my wants and do precisely what you want."

Neither expression, of course, is likely to make the other person happy. Indeed, both are likely to put the other person on the defensive. The latter expression, however, is likely to raise less defensiveness than the former. Others cannot argue with us about what we feel. If we feel it, we feel it. We have the right to our opinion, but this is quite different from telling someone that he is inconsiderate and thoughtless.

It is not easy to talk without using forms of the verb "to be." Indeed, the authors are not recommending that anyone seriously try to do so. We do maintain, however, that communication is less confrontative when we modestly stay within our own opinions rather than pontificate about the way things *really* are.

## Sending "I" Messages

Thomas Gordon suggests another way to reduce stressful encounters with others. He recommends sending "I messages" rather than "You messages."[9] People create a great deal of antagonism in others when they accuse them, and "you messages" are often accusatory. When we make statements such as "You are inconsiderate," "You don't listen," or "You are so loud with that horn that you distract me from my reading," we often cause the other person to become defensive and to argue about the charge.

Sending "I messages" tends to elicit a differing response. For one thing, "I messages" are softer than "You messages." "I feel as though my wishes and my opinions are not considered" may elicit a different response from a spouse or friend than does "You are inconsiderate." Similarly, saying "I don't feel as if you're hearing me" may trigger a somewhat more receptive response than will "You don't listen." Sending "I messages" forces us to use a more personalized, "feelingful" language. When we send "I messages," we do not make charges about others, we merely tell them how we are feeling.

We are likely to receive more favorable responses from others if we are careful not to needlessly offend them. If we charge others with thoughtlessness or malice, they are likely to focus on defending themselves rather than on the legitimacy of our requests. They may resist and refuse a request because they may perceive the situation to involve a contest of wills and feel the need to refuse our requests to prove that they are not doormats to be stepped on. This contest can be avoided if we merely report our *feelings* rather than lecture others regarding their behavior.

Forcing our wills upon others with rough and insulting commands creates growing resentment in others. Such bullying communication engenders foot-dragging or, worse yet, a form of psychological guerilla warfare from others. Respectful requests couched in "I messages" are less likely to be perceived as a contest of wills, and the other person can now oblige us without losing self-respect. The use of "I messages" results in interpersonal gain, even in situations where we clearly have the right to demand compliance. The other person knows that a respectful request contains a command, but in this softer form, the command is more readily obeyed. Consider this request: "John, I'm having trouble explaining to the plant manager why it is necessary for you to be late so often. I'd appreciate it if you would take whatever precautions are necessary to be on time." We are less likely to take offense at this request than if we are told "Damn it, John, I want you to be here on time. I've had about enough of your tardiness." Admittedly, there are times in which such bluntness may be appropriate, but when such bluntness is customary, we are likely to pay a considerable price for this indulgence of anger.

# Summary

Our relationships with others may be the most rewarding of human experiences or the source of enormous stress. Rewarding relationships do not just happen. They are *cultivated*. In spite of the immense importance of relationships, most persons spend little effort in analyzing what goes into good relationships and even less effort in learning skills that are necessary to enrich them. In this chapter we have highlighted attitudes and skills that play a significant role in creating rich social support networks across which we can spread the shock of stressful life events.

## ENDNOTES

1. W. K. Estes, "An Experimental Study of Punishment," *Psychological Monographs* 57, no.3 (1944), 263.

2. Kenneth B. Matheny and C. Edwards, "Academic Improvement Through an Experimental Classroom Management System," *Journal of School Psychology* 12 (1974): 222–32.

3. L. Z. Bloom, K. L. Coburn, and F. C. Pearlman, *The New Assertive Woman* (New York: Delacorte, 1975).

4. Manual J. Smith, *When I Say No, I Feel Guilty* (New York: Dial Press, 1975).

5. Jan Kelly and Barbara Winship, *I Am Worth It* (Chicago: Nelson Hall, 1979).

6. Smith, *When I Say No.*

7. Ibid.

8. Eric Berne, *Transactional Analysis in Psychotherapy* (New York: Grove Press, 1961).

9. Thomas Gordon, *Parent Effectiveness Training* (New York: Wyden, 1970).

# CHAPTER SIX

# THE BASICS OF CHANGE

Give me the strength to accept with serenity
the things that cannot be changed.
Give me the courage to change the things
that can and should be changed.
And give me the wisdom to distinguish one from the other.
——Saint Francis of Assisi

Controlling stress often requires significant changes in routines or habits. Making changes, however, is not easy, and motivation to change dies a slow death without a map to guide our efforts. Good intentions fade quickly when we blindly stumble in attempts to bring about personal change. Quite often we build up a head of steam for change only to watch it dissipate uselessly in self-recriminations and unenlightened false starts. We are able to harness this energy only when we develop a careful plan for change—a plan that anticipates and successfully deals with barriers to change encountered within ourselves and the environment. A convincing, detailed plan for personal change often awakens renewed hope, and hope unleashes enormous energy. In this chapter we will help the reader increase the motivation for personal change by anticipating barriers to change and by identifying key elements in any successful plan for change.

# Questioning the Need to Change

Most people are troubled by the conflicting desires to improve their lives on the one hand and to celebrate them on the other. At times we are inclined to follow the early Greeks in their worship of *arete*, or excellence, or the Hindus in their endless search for perfection. At other times we become weary at the mere thought of such seemingly neurotic striving and conclude that life is for celebrating, not for changing.

How can we continue to strive for improvement and yet accept ourselves as we are? Self-acceptance is the first requirement for good mental health. The belief that we *should* be perfect leads to discontent with ourselves and others. Hugh Prather said, "My day has become a fraction happier ever since I realized that nothing is exactly the way I would like it to be. This is simply the way life is—and there goes one battle I don't have to fight anymore."[1]

This is the dilemma between doing and being. This dilemma is clearly represented in the themes of two pieces of modern literature— Richard Bach's *Jonathan Livingston Seagull* and James Kavanaugh's *Celebrate the Sun*. Bach's seagull and Kavanaugh's pelican share with the reader their competing views of the purpose of life.

The seagull is bent on defying conventional standards of acceptable performance in his pursuit of death-defying feats and perfect speed. All his waking hours are devoted to straining his muscles to climb higher and higher, to dive faster and faster, and to soar with blinding speed. While others are content to perch on the rocks and lazily spear the fish along the shoreline, Jonathan Livingston Seagull constantly struggles to improve his aeronautical skills.

Kavanaugh's pelican, Harry Langendorf Pelican, spent his youth, like Jonathan, in quest of excellence and leadership and taught his offspring likewise. One day his son challenges him to a contest to see who can dive the swiftest. The son's wings proved too feeble to lift him out of the dive, and he plunges to his death upon the ocean's surface. The pelican grieves over the tragedy, reacts against his earlier perfectionism, and subsequently begins to accept life with its imperfections.

By examining passages from each of the two books, we are able to see more clearly their competing value systems.

| JONATHAN | HARRY |
|---|---|
| As a seagull it took us a hundred years to get the idea that our purpose for living is to find perfection and to show it forth. | It is not important to be perfect pelicans. We want to be happy pelicans. To always strive is never to be satisfied. We can celebrate the sun. |
| I just want to know what I can do in the air and what I can't, that's all. The gull sees farthest who flies highest. | I only fly as high as I want to. I enjoy being here together. We have sad times and good times, tragedy and joy; whatever it is, we will have made it so. |
| Why is it so hard to convince a gull that his life is free and that he can prove it for himself if he'll just spend time practicing? | I want to know my friends, to enjoy them. And I want to enjoy myself. |
| You didn't die, did you? In death you manage to change your level of consciousness rather abruptly. | I will miss you. I love you so. Maybe that's what death is—missing someone. |
| Heaven is being perfect. You will begin to touch heaven in the moment that you touch perfect speed. Perfection doesn't have limits.[2] | I have enjoyed my life, flying along the shore, sitting quietly on the rocks, feeling the wind lift me into the air, tasting the fresh fish, seeing the sun everyday—and loving you, loving you so much[3.] |

The values of *both* Jonathan and Harry have appeal. Like Jonathan, we are at times drawn to the perfect—to the ultimate in self-development—and sense a gnawing discontent with any incompleteness. But, like Harry, at other times we find peace in accepting less demanding views of ourselves. Each position has its assets and its liabilities. The drive for perfection, like the search for the Holy Grail, can be exhilarating, but it also has its liabilities. In some cases it may create an insatiable thirst capable of driving us mad. In other cases it may signal a kind of brittleness, a discontent with anything other than the *perfect* accomplishment of difficult goals and an inability to celebrate approximations of our goals. Self-acceptance suggests a less feverish, less militant approach to life, but it may also lead to narcissistic smugness.

Archibald MacLeish wrote that modern Americans believe that whatever *can* be done *should* be done.[4] This worship of change for change's sake is likely to bend the human condition all out of shape. Often, it is more sensible to accept ourselves than to seek to change ourselves. The

Indian mystic Jiddu Krishnamurti suggested that efforts to change are often counterproductive:

> Forget the ideal, and be aware of what you are. Do not pursue what *should* be, but understand what *is*. The understanding of what you actually are is far more important than the pursuit of what you *should* be. Why? Because in understanding what you are there begins a spontaneous process of transformation, whereas in becoming what you think you should be there is not change at all.[5]

Most crucial is a sense of personal control. Choosing *not* to change may indicate as much self-control as choosing to change. Yet, while most people would benefit from greater self-acceptance, most people also have traits and habits that they seriously want to change, but do not know how. Furthermore, self-resignation from feelings of helplessness is emotionally crippling, whereas self-acceptance that comes from a reappraisal of the hurtfulness of the trait or behavior in question and the cost of making the change may contribute to a sense of being in control.

In preparing for change, three questions require consideration:

- Can the situation be changed?
- What will it cost to change it?
- And *how* can it be changed?

# Can the Situation Be Changed?

Some situations *cannot* be changed. We sometimes find ourselves caught up in human predicaments, common life straits imposed by our human limitations. These predicaments are part of the human condition and cannot be escaped. If we try to escape them rather than to cope appropriately with them, we merely create additional problems for ourselves.

## Human Predicaments

Erich Fromm suggested that many predicaments are occasioned by the unique position of the human being in the animal kingdom.[6] People are the only animals capable of self-objectification. People alone are able to piece together a self-concept. Their self-awareness is an endowment that follows from their position atop the phylogenetic scale. The human brain contains an astounding associative network. Each of the thirteen billion or so neurons housed in it are capable of up to sixty thousand connections. The brain's potential associations, then, are greater in number than the total combinations allowable by the celestial bodies in the known universe.

With this unique information storage and retrieval system, sometimes referred to as the biocomputer, people are able to think in terms of past, present, and future; to engage in mental trial and error; to objectify themselves; and even to conceive of their own deaths. In addition to these remarkable mental gymnastics, the advanced brain makes it possible to experience anxiety, guilt, and loneliness.

As exhilarating as self-awareness may be, it nevertheless contributes to a sense of separateness and alienation. Lesser animals never experience this in the poignant manner in which humans feel it. Humans seem to know that they have cut the umbilical cord and are now *on their own*. They alternately whimper dependently and then rail against the new-found freedom. They spend their days seeking a substitute for the instantaneous and effortless gratification afforded by their earlier interauterine existence. Some appear willing to give up their birthrights to freedom in exchange for a return to the painless paradise of the womb. Metaphorically speaking, when Adam and Eve ate of the Tree of Knowledge, and thus developed self-awareness, they were expelled from paradise. They had severed the umbilical cord that connected them to the rest of nature.

Self-awareness creates difficulties that cannot be solved. Separation resulting from the inability to be everywhere at once cannot be solved. Grief caused by the loss of a loved one cannot be solved. Concern for survival cannot be solved. Growing old cannot be solved. Many times having cancer or suffering an amputation cannot be solved. None of these conditions has solutions. They are inescapable human predicaments with which we must learn to cope. Treating them as though they were problems that could be solved is a serious mistake.

Other human predicaments are created by personal value systems. In order to change certain situations, it may be necessary to violate these values. Once a client complained to one of the authors that she was living with her husband in quiet desperation. She saw herself as vibrant, outgoing, and somewhat experimental, and he as quite the opposite. He was a good, responsible man, but his needs for intimacy were minimal. She felt herself drying up psychologically for lack of touch, warmth, and sharing. She had approached him many times about her needs, but each time he had become embarrassed and changed the subject.

Although divorce had crossed her mind many times, she did not feel free to do so. Her personal values effectively thwarted her in taking such action. She was a deeply committed Roman Catholic and respected the Church's proscription against divorce. Furthermore, it was important to her to think of herself as a kind, considerate person who could never hurt a husband who did not deserve such treatment. Moreover, she thought of herself as a loving, responsible mother who would not cause suffering for her children in order to meet her selfish needs. These values were as effective as steel bands in restraining her from seeking a divorce. She was caught in a human predicament stemming from her own value system. While trapped in a relationship that offered little intimacy, she was unwilling to terminate the relationship because she had calculated the cost in terms of her personal values. This predicament was not to be solved; the answer lay in coping as cleverly as possible.

## Cultural Doublebinds

Cultural prescriptions for behavior are not always sane. The keen observer can usually spot within any society certain cultural prescriptions that are paradoxical. One that is common to American culture is the command, "Be spontaneous!" The point is that we cannot behave spontaneously while responding to a command. American culture is replete with examples of doublebinds, many of which are thrust upon children by their parents. Some parents are not content merely to force their children to do what they require of them; they also demand evidence that the youngsters want to do it. At an amusement park, a disconcerted mother was overheard saying to her child, "I spent a lot of money getting you in here, and you're going to enjoy it if I have to beat you within an inch of your life!" Dan Greenburg offers the following example of another kind of parental doublebind in his book, *How to Be a Jewish Mother*: "Give your son, Marvin, two sport shirts as a present. The first time he wears one of them, look at him sadly and say in your Basic Tone of Voice: 'The other one you didn't like?'"[7]

American women are frequently caught in doublebind demands. While they are exhorted to execute fully their maternal duties by devoting themselves for years to the rearing of their offspring, at the same time they are scolded for clinging to the security of the home and urged to move out into the work world and assume their obligations. If the mother chooses to remain in the home with her children, she is likely to feel insipid, immature, and fearful. If she returns to the work world, she may see herself as a selfish, heartless, neglectful parent. In such doublebinds she is damned if she does and damned if she doesn't. She will find little salvation from her dilemma until she recognizes the insolvable nature of the doublebind.

## The Wisdom to Know the Difference

How do we distinguish a *difficulty* with which we must cope from a *problem* that can be solved? No simple rule works in every case, but there are a few clues we can use to diagnose the difference. We are usually dealing with a difficulty—

- If the trouble stems from biological limitations, such as shortness, unpleasant physical features, or congenital deformities.
- If the only recognizable alternatives involve a clear violation of important values.
- If the locus of responsibility for resolving the issue lies within others. If others must change in order to make our lives better, or if we are making unreasonable demands on others in order to meet our needs, we are likely to be dealing with a difficulty with which we must cope rather than solve.

On the other hand, if we are looking to ourselves to exercise options available to us, we are likely to be dealing with a problem that can be solved.

## Coping Versus Combating

The noted stressologist Hans Selye points out that the body deals with toxins either syntoxically or catatoxically.[8] A *syntoxic* reaction tranquilizes the offended tissue and creates a state of passive tolerance or peaceful coexistence with the toxin. On the other hand, a *catatoxic* reaction triggers enzymes that attack it. These same reactions are appropriate in dealing with psychological stressors. It is appropriate to combat some stressors to try to eliminate them, but others must be coped with syntoxically.

# What Will It Cost Me to Change?

Before embarking on an extensive program of self-change, ask yourself, "Do I really want to change?" Perhaps more appropriately, ask, "How *badly* do I want to change?" There is an old Spanish proverb that says, "Take what you will, but pay for it," and it is a wise person who realizes that everything has its price. We cannot take responsibility for a new course of action without first assessing the costs involved.

Therapists quickly learn that the majority of clients are ambivalent about changing. They are miserable, confused by their symptoms, and therefore, driven to seek relief. They are even willing to expose their weaknesses to the therapist and to pay dearly for the privilege, and yet most clients are still ambivalent about changing. However self-defeating their symptoms may be in the long run, they tend to furnish some kind of immediate release from pent-up emotions. Consequently, clients sense that they must give up the familiar, immediate sources of nourishment in the hope that they will find more substantial sources within themselves and others—a risky business. For this reason clients secretly embrace their symptoms as old friends and resist change in spite of having come for therapy. The existential therapist Sheldon Kopp says the client often "prefers the security of known misery to the misery of unfamiliar insecurity."[9] The therapist knows that no genuine progress will be experienced until the client is willing to loosen the grasp, to lift anchor, and to suffer through the change. We are all very much this way. We sense that growth does not come easily, that the old with its security must give way to allow for the new.

Seldom do significant personal changes occur without psychic pain of some sort. Perhaps the benchmark of a growing maturity is the willingness to suffer. Because being responsible for ourselves is frightening, we often look for parental substitutes to spare us the ordeal. We give away our freedom to spouses, bosses, or friends. They become our parents, our psychological authority figures. *We* have put *them* in charge of *our* lives. We now must ask permission of them for behavioral options which were clearly ours in the first place.

Depression often is the price of turning our backs on self-direction and self-creation. It seems healthier to suffer the pain that comes from pursuing growth than the self-recrimination that follows retreat from growth and self-direction. In urging us to have the courage to take charge, Kopp wrote: "All . . . important decisions must be made on the basis of insufficient data. It is enough if a man accepts his freedom, takes his best shot, does what he can, faces the consequences of his acts, and makes no excuses."[10]

Sometimes confession constitutes a request for permission. If we announce that we have a low boiling point, we may in reality be asking permission to explode when it suits our purpose. This is a way of asking not to be held accountable for behavior.

A man who attempts to talk his wife into an open-marriage relationship so that he can have an affair with impunity is in effect seeking her permission. He wants to make her responsible for his behavior. He could have an affair without her permission, but then he would have to be responsible for the consequences. Responsibility involves accepting the consequences before committing an act. And since responsibility is so frightening, we are often ambivalent about making even those changes that seem desirable.

## Destroying to Create

The Hindus created the first systematic approach to personal change. They refer to God in three primary forms: Brahma, the creator; Vishnu, the preserver; and Shiva, the destroyer. It often puzzles Westerns that Shiva, who is a destroyer, should be deserving of worship. But with their total commitment to personal growth, the Hindus learned early that the old sometimes must be destroyed before the new can be created. New life is always built upon the rubble of the old.

Similar processes operate within the human body, which replaces

**Exhibit 6-1.** The Life Cycle Maintained by the Hindu Trinity

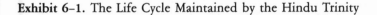

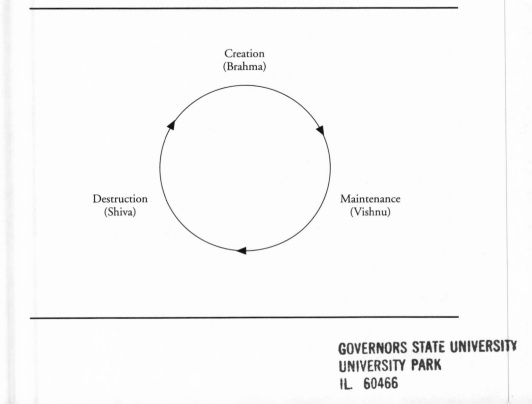

Creation
(Brahma)

Destruction
(Shiva)

Maintenance
(Vishnu)

itself completely every seven years. The complementary processes of catabolism and anabolism are constantly at work. It is necessary to break down the old atomic patterns of the organic fuel through catabolism before the atoms can be reassembled through anabolism into life forms. Life-death, death-life—the cycle goes on endlessly. Each is necessary to the existence of the other. We must lift a foot off the secure rung below in order to climb a ladder. And we must give up some incomplete and self-defeating present comforts in order to gain the opportunity to try for more fulfilling life adjustments.

Growth or self-renewal sometimes requires the destruction of old relationships and old self-images. Some people are locked into unsatisfying and unfulfilling marital relationships out of fear. Such people may engage in obsequious behavior in order to maintain a relationship. They may suffer psychological and physical abuse rather than give up even the threadbare security of a demeaning relationship. Although divorce is often counterproductive, it can sometimes purchase the possibility of needed self-redefinition—a heavy price, but sometimes one that is better than the readjustment required to maintain an exploitative relationship.

An ancient Chinese saying warns that a crisis signals both danger and opportunity. Sometimes crises destroy old relationships that have been maintained at great expense to ourselves. We may have held on to these relationships only out of fear that we would be unable to form more satisfying ones.

## Playing Blind and Deaf

Much stress derives from behaviors dictated by inadequate models. Our insecurity and need for control leads us to fashion rigid views of who we are and how things work. The emotional satisfaction from "knowing" causes us to prefer being "right" over being happy. Buddhists have long maintained that misery comes from ignorance.

Unrealistic views of ourselves and the world result in a blind-and-deaf approach to the world. Everything, both animate and inanimate, is a kind of broadcasting station that is constantly sending signals—trying to tell us about itself. The signals furnish vital information that can equip us to respect, enjoy, and use our world. Narrow, unrealistic views cause us to experience ourselves and others in incomplete ways. We only pick up those aspects of the signal or message that are in accord with existing impressions.

The Hindus call this illusion, *maya*. Maya furnishes a poor base from which to make life decisions; consequently, people often fail. Failure, in turn, causes us to become even more defensive in perceptual contacts with the world, and the resulting narrowness of perception leads to even more unrealistic views of self and the world. The antidote? *Shiva.* Destroy the old, unrealistic self-image in order to open up to more complete signals.

Swiss psychologist Jean Piaget suggests that there are two invariant functions by which we adjust to the world: assimilation and accommodation.[11] We assimilate a new experience when we force its characteristics to fit within a category or concept we have already hammered out. We accommodate when we force changes in ready-made concepts to make them conform better to reality. An old concept may be enlarged or enriched, or a new one may be required. It is easier to assimilate than to accommodate. We are reluctant to change ready-made structure, and, consequently, we often ignore significant signals from experiences in order to assimilate these experiences within old concepts. The more we do this, the more we contribute to maya, that unrealistic and unworkable view of ourselves and the world.

When people force new experiences into old frames, they grow detached from them. A general boredom sets in. Life becomes a rerun, and they just sit and stare. Such persons crave excitement because they consistently have ignored data that does not fit nicely into their ready-made models of how things work. William Blake said, "If the doors of perception were cleansed, everything would appear to man as it is, infinite. For man has closed himself up till he sees only through narrow chinks of his cavern."[12] And Arthur Koestler in *The Sleepwalkers* states: "Every creative act involves . . . a new innocence of perception, liberated from the cataract of accepted beliefs."[13] And Shunryu Suzuki observes that when our eyes are *open*, "the earth is its own magic."[14]

Sometimes we are forced by failure to change unrealistic views. Excellent examples are the people who are fired from a job only to find that they move into a much more rewarding position they might not otherwise have sought. Failure, therefore, need not always be viewed as tragedy; failure can indeed contribute to the growth cycle if it prompts the destruction of inadequate frames of reference and stimulates the construction of more adequate ones.

# How Do We Change?

Once we have resolved to change, we must settle on a strategy for bringing about the change. Very often we despair of changing, since we believe that all available solutions have been tried. Unfortunately, this happens when we have locked ourselves into a limiting class of solutions by unnecessary assumptions regarding what can and cannot be done about the problem behavior.

## Removing Perceptual Barriers to Change

Fisch, Weakland, and Segal point out that some problems are unresolvable as long as we limit ourselves unnecessarily to certain classes of solutions. In such cases we pointlessly try over and over again to make these solutions work. We operate with a kind of tunnel vision and fail to see more creative possibilities.[15]

The need for removing such perceptual barriers can be convincingly demonstrated with the nine dot problem.[16] The reader is asked to connect the nine dots shown in Exhibit 6–2 using only four straight lines and without lifting the pencil from the paper or retracing any lines.

Most of us struggle at length with this problem because we operate within a limiting mind-set. We assume that the dots define a square, and that we must not violate the sides of that square to find the solution. Once having made this assumption, we repeatedly try differing combinations of four lines with the same inevitable result: one of the dots always remains unconnected.

The solution of this problem is possible only when we destroy our old mind-set. Then, and only then, are we free to extend the lines beyond the imaginary "square," which was, after all, only in our minds. (The instructions for the problem made no mention of a square.) This problem parallels so many problems that persist only because of limiting, nonfunctional, self-imposed assumptions. (The solution to the Nine-dot Problem appears at the end of the chapter.) Limiting ourselves to an inadequate class of solutions is doubly hurtful, for it blinds us to other potential solutions and sometimes counterproductive efforts to resolve the problem result in making the problem worse.

## The Solution Is the Problem

Sometimes the actions we take to deal with stressors actually create additional stress for us. The husband who feels neglected by his wife

**Exhibit 6-2.** The Nine-dot Problem

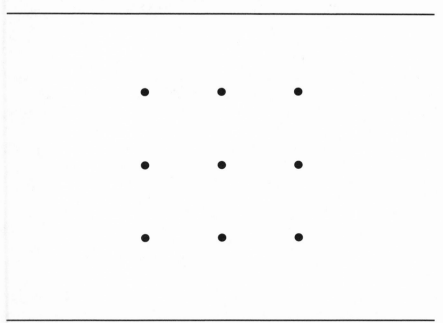

may demand attention to such an extent that she moves away from him. The more possessive he becomes of her time and attention, the more entrapped and consumed she feels. Consequently, she manufactures reasons for absenting herself from him. Thus, the very behaviors that he used to seek her attention cause her to ignore him in self-defense. His solution has become the problem.

A wife may be irritated by her husband's eternal pessimism and cynicism and may respond overly optimistically. He, in turn, may view her optimism as naive and attempt to moderate her views by repeatedly drawing her attention to the seamy, distressful side of life. The more they work on each other's problems, the greater the psychological distance between them becomes. As with so many marital and family problems, the solution has become the problem, and giving up on the problem sometimes makes things better. Sometimes couples rediscover their attraction for each other after they decide to get a divorce. At this point each gives up on the other, stops trying to make the other over, and the spontaneity and attractiveness sometimes returns.

One client, a middle-aged woman, complained that her husband was sabotaging her efforts to discipline their fifteen-year-old daughter. She had accumulated much resentment toward him and worried greatly about the fate of her daughter. Her husband believed she was too hard on the daughter, and he often protected her from his wife's ire. Concluding that it would be necessary for her to perform the disciplinary tasks of both father and mother, the mother became increasingly severe with the daughter. The more she disciplined her, however, the more the husband felt it necessary to erode her power base, and the more the husband and daughter aligned themselves against the mother.

A break in this disastrous cycle came when the mother realized that her behavior was actually contributing to the growing defection of both daughter and husband. She shared her insight with them and announced that she was delivering over to the husband the task of disciplining the daughter, since her efforts had clearly been self-defeating. She withdrew from potential conflicts, even when it pained her greatly. In the ensuing vacuum, the husband was forced to change his role with regard to his daughter, and consequently, the previous alliance between husband and daughter loosened. The woman wisely refrained from "I told you so" scenes, and instead offered support to the husband when he shared his difficulty in properly managing the daughter. As a result of this paradoxical technique, the relationship between wife and husband steadily improved.

When you are at an impasse in your relationship with others, it is a good idea to back off, lower the attendant emotion, and ask "What is going on here?" Perhaps you will discover that the more you try to resolve the issue the more damaging it becomes. In such cases *more of the same* will only make matters worse. Not understanding this, we are often caught up in interpersonal games without end, and the harder we play the more we get punished.

In summary, it is often helpful to change the mind-set with which a problem is approached. If we can recognize the limiting assumptions that have been made about classes of solutions, we can open ourselves to more creative approaches.

## Defining the Problem

From the foregoing discussion, we clearly see the importance of defining a problem properly. The first and most important step in designing a strategy for self-change is to state the problem openly enough to allow for competing classes of solutions. For example, the problem statement "How can I get into medical school with my C + undergraduate grade point average?" may be unnecessarily restrictive. It is possible that the motivation behind this question is the search for an occupation that will offer many of the same financial and social rewards that are derived from the practice of medicine. In this eventuality, the problem statement might more appropriately become, "How can I identify and gain entrance into some occupation that will provide a high degree of financial success and social esteem?" Even in this form the problem undoubtedly will be difficult to solve, but gaining entrance to medical school with a C + average is all but impossible and, moreover, is unnecessary if the second question is a more accurate statement of the problem.

Similarly, the problem "How can I get my spouse to become interested in tennis?" may be too restrictive. Perhaps a more apt statement of the problem would be: "How can I play tennis more often without feeling guilty about the time I am away from the family and without causing my spouse to become angry with me?" This broader statement allows for a larger number of potential solutions. We may never be able to interest our spouses in the game, regardless of all the inducements we propose. Nevertheless, there are many classes of potential solutions to the second, more broadly stated, problem statement.

A problem statement must also be *specific* enough to be attackable. Vague complaints must be translated into specific behaviors. The problem statement "I'm depressed and nothing seems to turn me on" in its present form is attackable only through medication. Upon further reflection, the statement may become: "I've tried and tried to screw up the courage to ask a classmate for a date, but I'm afraid that she might turn me down, and, on the other hand, I'm afraid she might accept because I don't know how to talk to women alone." This more specific statement is attackable on two fronts. We can attack the inhibiting self-talk, which says, "If she turned me down, that would be crushing — absolutely terrible. My ego couldn't cope with that!" And we can attack his lack of social skills.

A problem statement should lead to reasonable goals for accomplishment. People who feel inadequate often overreact and make perfectionistic demands on themselves. When perfectionism is overcompensation for perceived weaknesses, it is merely a cop out, a mind trip we run on ourselves to delay starting the hard work required to change. If we assume that the only goals worth pursuing are virtually impossible to achieve, then we can be excused for not trying at all. To dream the impossible dream may be noble and romantic, but it is hardly practical or likely to accomplish a desired change.

Gary Latham and Edwin Locke found that successful people tend to set moderate, rather than perfectionistic, goals.[17] Since we borrow strength from past accomplishments for present endeavors, we are likely to bog down from insufficient motivation if we set goals that require extremely difficult performances.

In summary, we are ready to plan strategies for personal change only after the problem has been stated in a way that allows for as many solutions as possible, in a way that is specific enough to be attackable, and in a way that is modest enough to be achievable.

## Focusing on Behavior

Whenever we experience performance failures, we often accuse ourselves of being weak, lazy, or incompetent. Such name-calling, however, does little to correct the behavior. It is far better to question the adequacy of our behavior in these cases than to attack our characters. If we describe a problem as "laziness" or "incompetence," there is no clear direction for pursuing a solution. Once we use such pejorative terms we close ourselves off to practical courses of action. Such terms result from sloppy thinking. It is better to define a problem in terms of behavior than in terms of traits. Rather than conclude that we are lazy, it may be better to say, if appropriate, "I have not yet located an approach to my work that seems likely to succeed, and, therefore, it's hard for me to be involved with it." This statement seems more helpful, for it may lead us to seek consultation from others or to try other new approaches.

The focus should be on replacement behaviors. Ask "What can I do differently that will help me to better cope with the situation?" If you experience stress from a failure to stand up for your rights, perhaps you should attend a workshop on assertiveness training or read books on the subject. If your study habits distress you, perhaps you should compare your habits with those of students who earn better marks. If you are stressed by your failure to get your children to do their chores, avoid the temptation to verbally attack yourself for your "incompetence" and, instead, focus attention on what you and the children are doing. Examine *what happens* when they do and do not perform the chores. Children sometimes condition a parent to give in by responding angrily and only half completing a task. If this is the case, you may wish to establish a rule that the children cannot play until their work is done. Obviously, any such move is attendant with hazards, but the point is that you should question your methods, *not your person.*

## Attention Directs the Energy Flow

Attention is a powerful tool for personal change. Directing attention to a behavior quite often affects the frequency of it. For this reason, drivers are instructed to direct their vision to the solid line along the right shoulder of the road when the lights of the approaching vehicle make it difficult to see. We are drawn toward the object of our attention. If drivers look at the lights of the oncoming vehicle, they are more likely to turn the nose of the car into its path.

The act of directing attention is equivalent to directing the flow of energy. Soviet experimentation with *Kirlian photography,* a lensless process of filming the electromagnetic field surrounding living bodies, underscores this principle quite strongly. Through Kirlian photography, Soviet researchers found that subjects are quite capable of influencing their electromagnetic fields through concentrated attention.[18] Thus, focusing attention on positive behaviors directs energy to them and makes them more likely to occur. Attending to a problem in a *constructive* manner is helpful on two accounts: it helps us to understand the conditions that trigger and maintain behavior, and it furnishes feedback on progress toward replacement behavior.

Very little, if any, behavior in one-celled life forms seems self-initiated. These life forms move only as a reaction to outside stimuli, and their relationship to the environment is basically reactive. A person's relationship to the environment, however, is much more complex and interactional. We are influenced by the environment, but we, in turn, influence it as well. Moreover, our behavior is quite often a response to internal stimulation, such as ideas, thoughts, beliefs, and images. If we are to change our behavior, then we must influence those stimulus conditions that govern it.

There are two classes of stimuli: those that precede the behavior, called *cues*, and those that follow behavior, called *consequences*. While both influence behavior, their functions are different. Cues are signals that prompt us either to avoid or to initiate a course of action, depending upon our previous experience with it. If the consequences of a behavior are perceived as pleasant, then cues previously associated with the behavior flash a green light for the behavior; if the consequences are disagreeable, then a red light is signalled. Consequent stimuli are stimuli coming after the behavior. They may be rewarding or punishing. Cues and consequences work together in controlling behavior.

## Changing the Cues

Cues are essential guides to behavior. Intelligent behavior requires both a repertoire of skillful responses and a sense of timing in the performance of these responses. It is highly useful to be able to express affection, but it is not always appropriate to do so. It is also useful to be able to express irritation and anger, but the cost of doing so may be dear if the situation is inappropriate. If we have been fortunate, our experiences have provided cues to assist in recognizing the conditions in which such responses are appropriate. Unfortunately, not all experiences prepare us to perform appropriately. Some childhood training may have taught inappropriate cues. For example, we may have learned to cower, fawn, or otherwise appear helpless when confronted by powerful people (parents or other adults). Some people learn to bellow and intimidate when they are in a situation where others control important resources.

The cues that trigger a child's responses may have been quite functional for a child, but these same cues are often inappropriate guides for adult behavior. A child mistreated by a malevolent, uncaring father may learn to respond cautiously and obsequiously in his presence. The father's presence, then, becomes a cue to trigger fearful, dependent behavior. Consequently, the child may experience these same behaviors as an adult. Worse yet, the tendency to defer may spread to other powerful figures reminiscent of the father. Although they have outlived their usefulness, these cues may continue to cause the person discomfort.

Since such cues often function more or less unconsciously in our lives, we may not know why we freeze emotionally or respond with cowardice, or why we cannot think straight or assert ourselves on certain occasions. We can discover the relationships between such cues and behavior by attending to situations immediately preceding the disliked behavior. A cigarette machine, a coffee break, or being in the presence of someone smoking may constitute a strong cue to smoke. The sight of a refrigerator, a cookie jar or, in many cases, a TV set may serve as a cue for eating. If we can identify such cues, we can try to avoid them or attempt to change their signal value.

The reader may remember the efforts of Odysseus, Homer's character, to avoid certain tempting cues for himself and his crewmen. It was the practice of the Sirens to lure passing seamen to their deaths with their enchanting calls. To avoid hearing the seductive Sirens, Odysseus commanded his men to fill their ears with beeswax and had himself tied to the mast. These precautions were maintained until the seamen were safely out of hearing range.

In a similar manner, we may choose to avoid certain cues that trigger undesirable behavior. Some time ago, one of the authors was interested in losing ten pounds. He analyzed his eating habits and concluded that during the daylight hours his intake of calories was actually less than the number required to maintain his weight. From 9:00 p.m. to 11:00 p.m., however, he ate continuously while watching television. He was often bored with the quality of the programming; consequently, he passed the hours pleasantly with the help of food. He decided to retire at 9:30 p.m. in order to avoid the nightly gorging. The plan worked splendidly, and he lost the ten pounds in fewer than six weeks. He successfully changed his behavior not by punishing the act of overeating, but by avoiding the stimuli that triggered it.

Behavior often is situation-specific, that is, it occurs *only* in certain situations. If we can identify these situations and avoid them or remove them, we can effectively reduce the behavior in question. Some time ago a youngster accused of being rebellious and disrespectful by a teacher was sent to one of the authors for counseling. He found that the boy behaved acceptably in other classrooms, a fact later confirmed by the principal. Moreover, the rebellious and disrespectful behavior always followed criticisms by the teacher of his personal grooming and sloppy handwriting. Upon learning this, the author decided that his real client was the teacher. He decided that the child's inappropriate behavior was, in fact, understandable in light of the teacher's criticisms of his person and handwriting. The author tactfully shared this observation with the teacher, who made a concerted effort thereafter to avoid such adverse criticism. The happy result was that the child's rebelliousness predictably subsided. In this case the cue was removed, and the triggered behavior disappeared.

It is not always possible to avoid or remove a triggering cue. In such cases it is sometimes possible to change the signal value of such cues, that is, to destroy a cue's ability to trigger the undesirable behavior. It was noted earlier that the cue derives its ability to trigger avoidance or approach from its association with rewarding or punishing consequences following behavior. One of the authors noted that his cat rubbed her fur across his legs and meowed loudly when he approached the refrigerator—provided she was hungry. The cat obviously had noticed that he went to the refrigerator before placing food in her dish. His approach to the refrigerator, then, had become a signal that something very good was about to happen. This cue then triggered the cat to meow and rub against his legs, which, it must have seemed to the cat, encouraged him to feed her. Indeed, the strategy often worked. In this example, the approach to the refrigerator cued the cat's behavior, which, in turn, cued the author's obliging response.

If a cue derives its power to trigger behavior from its association with the consequences of the behavior, then we can extinguish a cue by changing the perceived consequences of the behavior. If the author were to kick the cat each time he opened the refrigerator door, approaching the refrigerator would become a cue for the cat to scurry out of the room. His changed behavior would change the signal value of the cue by changing the resulting consequences. This would be an example of aversion therapy.

Aversion therapy is a somewhat questionable technique in behavior therapy. It has been used to treat drinking problems. Since the liquor bottle, liquor glass, and other paraphernalia associated with the habit are known to be cues for the act of drinking, the task of aversion therapy is to cause such paraphernalia to trigger a "stop drinking" response rather than a "drinking" one. Upon giving his consent, a client is wired so that a mildly disagreeable electrical current is directed to one of his fingers immediately following his movement toward such objects. The current stops when he moves away from the objects. This process is designed to cause these paraphernalia to trigger nondrinking rather than drinking behavior by changing their cue value.

## Changing the Consequences

It is also important to direct our attention to the consequences of our behavior. What happens after we get angry, cry, apologize or withdraw from an argument? We do what we get paid for. If we continue a behavior, even one that grieves us, it must be because at some level of awareness we perceive it to be rewarding. This concept is sometimes difficult to understand, for it seems that there are no rewards for some habits. How are we rewarded for the fit of anger that embarrasses, the flood of tears that makes us appear childish, or sickeningly compliant behavior in the face of demands by others? On cursory inspection such behaviors appear to hurt in every respect. Upon closer scrutiny, however, we may discover hidden rewards. The compliance that results in self-contempt may reduce the anxiety felt when we sense that confrontation is brewing. The tears that make us feel childish may bring the nurturing attention of people important to us. And the anger that embarrasses may intimidate others and cause them to allow us to have our way.

When self-defeating behavior is maintained by hidden rewards, the person may lack the motivation to change it. We authors at times have tried to help clients change behaviors only to find that they were inadequately motivated to change them. There were hidden purposes for the behavior, and these clients were unconsciously resisting change. When we discover that undesirable habits are reinforced by hitherto unrecognized consequences, we are free to search for more acceptable ways of serving the same end.

We sometimes despair of reforming our behavior because we believe our efforts are not likely to be rewarded. We may no longer express irritation when others violate our rights because the consequences of earlier efforts were perceived as being punishing. We may find it difficult to persist at homework assignments, because it may appear that past study efforts did little to improve grades. We may abandon efforts to get our children to do household chores because the resulting conflict was so unpleasant. We may have difficulty motivating ourselves to apply for a better job if previous efforts were perceived to be unsuccessful.

## Present Tense Explanations of Behavior

You will note that we have not recommended an extended pilgrimage into the distant past in order to understand your behavior. The authors believe that it generally is *not* cost-effective to devote considerable time to searching out the historical determinants of behaviors that need changing. A simplistic but somewhat surprising truth about the past is that it no longer exists! Only the *perception* of the past exists. The search for the past context out of which the troublesome behavior emerged often concludes with a curious admixture of fact and fiction. While understanding our perception of the past may be satisfying, at worst it may furnish us with ready-made villains to blame for our problem. We may use these villains to excuse ourselves from accepting personal responsibility for our behavior.

While the past-oriented "why" used in the question "Why have I become the way I am?" may or may not be particularly helpful, an understanding of the present-oriented "why" is absolutely essential for designing any change strategy. It draws attention to present factors, to cues and consequences that make the behavior more likely.

The importance of focusing clearly on the present-oriented "why" can be seen in the following case. Ann sought therapy because of her inadequacy in dealing with her home situation. Her husband Bob had brought his mother to live with them following a long hospitalization for a broken hip. The mother-in-law always seemed to be in the way. Ann and her mother-in-law clashed often over the manner in which the children were being reared. Ann thought her mother-in-law overindulged the children. She constantly gave them money, and while Ann did not confront her over this, she did make the children return the money. The mother-in-law sided with the children in their rebellion at going to bed, but Ann ignored her and nagged the children until they finally went to bed. In many other situations, the mother-in-law greatly aggravated Ann's difficulties in handling the children. Whenever Ann complained about the situation, Bob became furious. Ann believed that it was bad for the children to see their father so angry with her; consequently, she would quickly apologize and avoid bringing up the issue again.

This situation could be approached without any investigation whatsoever of Ann's past. The problem could be viewed as her failure to assert herself effectively with her husband and mother-in-law. Even as she attempted to assert herself, she retreated under fire. We merely needed to identify the cues triggering her retreat and the consequences that followed. There were at least three cues that triggered her retreat: (1) her belief that the children should not see their father in a state of rage, (2) the angry retort of her husband, and (3) the fear that it aroused. The rewarding consequences of her retreat were a lessening of her husband's anger and a subsequent reduction in her fear. The punishing consequences of her retreat were the continuing interference of the mother-in-law and the self-contempt that Ann experienced. By becoming aware of the nature of her behavior, Ann was able to deal more effectively with the situation.

## Sketching the Context

We have seen the importance of understanding the context within which undesirable behavior is likely to occur. We recognize the importance of cues for initiating the behavior and consequences for maintaining it. We also realize that cues and consequences can consist of thoughts and beliefs as well as the behaviors of others. If we wish to discourage undesirable behavior, we must attempt to eliminate the cues and consequences associated with it; and if we are to encourage replacement behaviors, we must attempt to establish a context within which it is most likely to occur. The following is a greatly abbreviated example of

## Context for Overeating

| Source | Cues | | Consequences |
|---|---|---|---|
| External Environment | *Seeing appealing sweets.* *Viewing TV in the late evening.* *Seeing others snacking.* *Drinking alcohol.* | O V E R E A | *The playful, endorsing comments of others about how much I eat.* *Wife's obvious pleasure with my hearty appetite for her food.* |
| Internal Environment | *Mentally searching for pleasure to counter boredom.* *Telling myself that I deserve a reward for working hard.* *Conditioning — habitual eating.* | T I N G | *The intrinsic pleasure of eating itself.* *The feeling of being full and satisfied.* |

## Context for Calorie-Conscious Eating

| Source | Cues | | Consequences |
|---|---|---|---|
| External Environment | *Activities that keep me interested.* *Being physically active.* *Lively conversations with others.* *Meditation or Yoga.* | U N D E R | *Occasional comments from others endorsing my weight loss.* *Clothing looks better on me.* *No pinching of stomach fat when sitting.* *The lower reading on the weight scales.* *Walk longer with less effort.* |
| Internal Environment | *Telling myself that I am getting my weight under control.* *Telling myself that less weight will mean less strain on the heart.* *Telling myself that I will look better in my clothes.* *Telling myself that being a little hungry is a sign of thinning down.* | E A T I N G | *Food tastes better.* *Feel lighter on my feet when walking.* *Clothing fits me less tightly.* *Being proud of myself for my self-discipline.* |

the contextual analysis of the overeating behavior of a client seen by one of the authors.

In order to encourage an eating regimen that would help the client lose weight, the author-therapist, along with the client, constructed a desirable context for more restrained eating. An abbreviated version of this effort appears on the following page. The purpose of identifying the context for behavior is to allow for greater control over it. In this case it meant trying to eliminate cues and consequences that encouraged overeating and to arrange conditions that would encourage more calorie-conscious eating. While it is difficult to control the reactions of others, there usually are many things we can do ourselves to influence our behavior. As a result of the first contextual analysis the client was encouraged to

- remove sweets from the home and to avoid shopping for groceries when hungry.
- engage in more active pursuits in the evening to counter the boredom from long hours of TV viewing.
- drink less alcohol inasmuch as it rendered him less intent on controlling his eating.
- eat dinner later in the evening and to retire earlier in order to discourage late-night eating.
- enlist his wife's support.
- announce his intentions to lose weight to others in order to put additional pressure on himself to succeed.
- constantly edit his thinking—to eliminate self-talk, which suggested that eating high-caloric foods was a just reward for working hard, and in its place to tell himself that he is getting his weight under control, that he will look better in his clothing, that he will be able to move with less effort, that he will present a better image to others, that he will have more self-respect, and the like.

## Making Rewards Conditional

After we have properly defined a behavior and carefully attended to cues and consequences, we must plan to provide rewards for any intended change. We should do this on the same basis that it is done in business and industry. The rewards must be conditional, that is, they must be made contingent upon the desired performance.

The self-administration of rewards is a tricky matter. It is always possible to cheat, for who will know? We can partly take care of this problem by making public our intentions. Most people do better if they put pressure on themselves by informing others of their goals and progress. Nevertheless, under the most stringent precautions, there are still opportunities for cheating. And there is ultimately no foolproof antidote for this.

There are, however, some ways to inhibit cheating. Some rewards, for example, lose their meaning when self-administered. What real gain is there in taking money out of one pocket and placing it in another? Money is an ineffective reward under such circumstances. There is one way, however, in which money can be a meaningful reward. That is when we give a significant sum to a trusted friend to be returned in agreed-upon amounts, provided we meet our goals. The money will be even more rewarding if the contract carries the proviso that it will be sent to some organization that violates our values if we fail to meet the goals. This plan worked beautifully for a doctoral student who had difficulty finishing his dissertation.

There are four basic classes of rewards: (1) tangibles, such as money, food or other objects; (2) social attention, such as compliments or expressions of affection; (3) enjoyable activities; and (4) feedback regarding progress. In the authors' experience, the last two classes of rewards are more useful than the first two in self-administered programs. Money and other tangibles are not usually rewarding when self-administered—for reasons already discussed. If compliments and expressions of affection are freely given by significant others, they are very motivating; indeed, they are among the most powerful of all rewards when given freely and spontaneously. Given at our request, however, they appear contrived and forced and are less effective.

Favorite activities used as rewards for behavior often work. A game of tennis, a few hours for loafing, an hour or two at the piano, going to the theater, and taking a trip are only a few of the possibilities. Such activities serve as rewards if we engage in them *only after reaching a goal*. First lose the excess weight, then take the trip. First do the required reading, then off to the tennis courts. First do the yoga exercises, then watch TV. Moreover, if such activities are to be rewarding, we must shut ourselves off from them at all other times. If we are already watching TV extensively, further viewing is unrewarding. If we play tennis several days a week, one more game is not likely to be sufficiently rewarding. In fact, it is wise to wean ourselves off any activity for a reasonable period before attempting to use it as a reward.

The most natural of all self-administered rewards is feedback regarding our progress. Very often people who attempt self-change programs tire of other rewards, but continue to value feedback. Without feedback virtually no progress is made. While feedback sometimes comes from others in the form of praise or criticism, feedback can also take the form of records that reflect progress.

## Finding the Starting Line

We need to know where both starting and finishing lines are before progress can be measured. If we have stated a problem specifically, the finish line, or goal, will be clearly in focus. It is also helpful in measuring progress to know where we started. One of the authors once had a client who refused to weigh herself before starting a diet. She said that she knew she was grossly overweight and did not want to punish herself by climbing on the scales. She managed to lose a modest amount of weight, but she was never quite certain how much. This kind of fuzziness about a starting line is usually discouraging, and it makes it difficult to know how well a plan is succeeding.

There are many ways of getting a reading on the frequency of a behavior. If we are trying to lose weight, then we can measure pounds, calories ingested, or snacks eaten. If we are trying to stop smoking, we can measure the number of cigarettes smoked in a twenty-four-hour period, the number of hours in the day in which we did not smoke, or even the length of time spent smoking. If we are trying to become more outgoing, we can measure the number of times during the day that we initiate conversation with others or the amount of time spent in the company of others.

## The Taste of Success

Few things are as rewarding as noting progress toward personal goals. The expression "Nothing succeeds like success" is particularly true in self-change programs. Feedback or knowledge of results, then, is crucial to personal change. It is for this reason that we are encouraged to keep continuous records of progress. We are unable to keep accurate records unless the behavior has been specifically defined. We must be able to identify instances and noninstances of the desired behavior. Without such specificity, efforts to chart progress are likely to be grossly inexact.

The frequency and kind of records depend largely on the kind of behavior in question. As a rule, however, a full day is as long as we should go without some kind of evaluation or recording. When a behavior is very difficult to begin, more frequent recording may be necessary. The recording itself is often rewarding, as it provides immediate feedback. If we have to wait for long periods without feedback, there is a tendency for motivation to sag. Many educational psychologists think that the nine-week report card periods used by many schools have little to do with performance because this period is too long to motivate most students. Daily grades are much more likely to influence behavior.

One author recalls advising a second-grade teacher to place five non-reading boys on a self-instructional program especially designed for nonreaders. The materials had considerable appeal to the boys, and they were soon making noticeable progress. When the teacher was convinced that the program was working, she decided to give her attention to other students. Approximately three days after she withdrew her attention, the boys complained of disinterest in the materials. The teacher took renewed interest in their performance, and as a result, the boys resumed their progress at the task. The teacher had withdrawn her powerfully reinforcing attention too soon. Similarly, withdrawing attention from self-progress before the behavior becomes thoroughly habitual is often disastrous to the program. We must continue to monitor the behavior, to chart, to keep records, to endorse ourselves, and to keep our eyes on the goal.

We simply cannot hope to make serious progress toward our goals without feedback. If a program for change is working, then knowing about it increases our resolve to continue. If it is not, then knowing about it allows us to make necessary adjustments.

Plans for change often require adjustments when they are put into action. We may have anticipated a complete and perfect performance before it is likely, and we may need to accept instead some approximation to the full-blown performance. We may have planned for a desirable consequence that, in fact, turns out to be less desirable in reality. We may find we have defined the problem behavior so abstractly that there is difficulty monitoring it.

Still, the need to structure a program remains. Structure is an effective antidote for the generalized anxiety that can result from the overwhelming ambiguity of some situations. One of the authors often allows himself to become foolishly overcommitted. As a result, he sometimes grows increasingly nervous over deadlines. Upon such occasions, the resulting anxiety is immobilizing. He sits staring aimlessly, looking for opportunities to be distracted, and generally accomplishes nothing of importance. It is only when he structures his commitments that his anxiety is assuaged. If he stops the cycle by carefully defining the full scope of the responsibilities assumed, if he establishes real time constraints, and if he identifies the enabling steps necessary to accomplish these responsibilities, then—and only then—does he feel relief from the nagging uneasiness.

While it is true that a journey of a thousand miles starts from where we presently are, it is vital to know in which direction to drop the first foot. Establishing structure is tedious; it takes effort, and, for most people, it is not fun. Nevertheless, people seldom carry through on important assignments without a reasonable degree of direction or structure. This is particularly important in the beginning. We may have failed several times at trying to change behavior, and unless we have a well-defined, reasonably convincing plan, our present efforts are likely to suffer an early death for lack of sustaining motivation.

## Beginning Efforts

When we begin a new behavior, two observations are quite likely. It may seem to take a lot of effort to get the new plan off the ground, and the new behavior quite likely will seem unnatural. There is a principle in mutual fund investments called front-end loading. When first beginning an investment plan with many of these mutual funds, a disproportionate amount of the initial investment is taken for administrative fees. With later investments, the amount accruing to an account increases markedly. Self-change programs are similar. To get any behavior started to any noticeable degree may require substantial attention and effort. Later, the behavior can be maintained with a fraction of the initial effort. Many of us can recall the initial awkwardness of learning to drive an automobile. Each maneuver, such as depressing the clutch and shifting gears, at first completely absorbs our full attention. Later, however, a rhythm is established, and the most complex of tasks flows as a simple, effortless performance.

People often discourage themselves from adopting new behaviors by saying such things as, "This is ridiculous! It's just not me. I feel like I'm just acting." But in reality, who is the real you or me? Behaviors that now seem natural were themselves awkward initially. Behaviors can be *naturally* good or *naturally* bad. We often attempt change because we conclude that a *natural* behavior is simply not functional. Swinging a golf club as we swing a baseball bat may feel quite natural to the beginner, but the trajectory of the ball hit this way often indicates that the swing is nonfunctional. The more we perform a new behavior, the more natural it will become.

## Effects of Time and Practice

Considerable time and practice are necessary for eliminating old responses and becoming used to new ones. Too often, a person develops an unrealistic time frame within which to accomplish a change. While it is only human nature to want to do something and get it over with, most habits are highly resistant to change and sometimes return spontaneously after we think we have eliminated them. Because of impatience people often fall prey to fad diets, easy-to-swallow mood changers, and weekend, personality-altering marathons. On the other hand, the best, time-tested formula for personal change looks like this:

$$Change: f \left\{ Motivation \times Plan\ for\ Change \times \frac{Practice}{Time} \right\}$$

Change is a function of motivation times planning times practice over an extended period of time. If any factor in the function is nonexistent (zero), the amount of change will be zero. Zero times anything is zero. Therefore the stronger the motivation, the more promising the program for change, the greater the practice, and the longer the program is maintained, the more significant the resulting change is likely to be.

## Rejecting Guilt

Once we are committed to a program of change, we should steadfastly resist the tendency to feel guilty over temporary backsliding. Guilt usually is nonproductive and depressing. It robs us of the motivation and energy necessary for change. Guilt often goes hand in hand with perfectionism. Both are usually counterproductive.

While it takes courage to embark on a journey to change old habits, it also takes courage to be *imperfect* along the way. Without tolerance for such imperfection, we can never stand the journey, because of its unpredictability and the possibility of failure.

The usual path of self-change is like the flight of a bird. There is some wing flapping, some climbing, and then some coasting. People, too, work hard at change for a while, and then tend to coast for a while. If we require perfectionism, we quit upon the first indication of backsliding or coasting. The Zen aphorism, "Gentle is the way," is good advice to counter these natural tendencies. We must be able to put backsliding into perspective. We must have a healthy respect for the difficulty involved in re-creation. The people who have the best chance for success are the ones who have come to accept themselves, whether climbing or coasting.

To counter the free-fall into collapsing, backsliders should remind themselves of some facts. Alan Marlatt maintains that, contrary to public opinion, the more often persons try to break a habit the *more likely* they are to do so![19] He criticizes the helping professions for focusing exclusively on efforts to assist addicts to withdraw from the use of abused substances without giving adequate attention to lapses in their abstinence. He maintains that a high percentage of substance abusers (for example alcoholics, smokers, overeaters) lapse, and these abusers must view these lapses as unfortunate but not devastating. He believes that conventional moral and medical views of addictive disorders undercut long-term maintenance by instilling all-or-nothing thinking. The moral view attributes addiction to a character flaw and the medical model to a disease beyond the person's control. Lapsing into further use of the addictive substance *for any period* is attributed to bad character by the moralists and to the continued presence of the disease for those subscribing to the medical model.

The all-or-nothing thinking implicit in the moral and medical positions leaves the abuser unable to distinguish a minor lapse from a major relapse. Consequently, the person may give up in the face of even minor lapses. Marlatt believes it is best to view addictive behaviors as resulting from overlearned habits, rather than from character disorders or underlying disease processes.[20] This view, when applied to alcoholics, has placed Marlatt in open conflict with Alcoholics Anonymous' view of alcoholism as a disease. He and his colleagues believe relapsing is most likely to occur during periods of emotional distress.[21] Consequently, they insist that any meaningful recovery program must sensitize addicts to those stressful situations most likely to trigger the relapse and must assist them beforehand to counter the thinking that promotes it.

A useful distinction needs to be made between stages of backsliding. The three stages are *lapsing*, *relapsing*, and *collapsing*. *Lapsing* refers to occasional slip-ups and should be viewed as a normal reaction to any effort to change. *Relapsing* is considerably more serious, as it refers to extended periods, usually weeks or months, wherein persons have dropped off efforts to change but still purport to make the change and believe that in time they will. *Collapsing* on the other hand signals a complete loss of morale wherein such persons feel helpless in the clutches of the habit. Marlatt maintains that lapsing is inevitable but relapsing is not. Relapsing is unfortunate but not all that unexpected. In this view it is more likely to become permanent only if persons hold moralistic or medical views of the basis for the addiction. Marlatt's relapse prevention model seeks to make relapses less likely by assisting persons in recovery to anticipate lapses and to avoid perfectionistic thinking that suggests "I've failed again; I might as well throw in the towel!" According to Marlatt's research of relapse situations, about 60 percent were determined by *intra*personal factors such as negative emotional states or urges and temptations. Roughly 40 percent of alcoholic relapses were determined by *inter*personal factors such as conflicts or social pressures. Kelly D. Brownell suggests that addicts should use a "forest ranger" metaphor in viewing their work in withdrawing. Their first task is to prevent fires (lapses), and their second is to put the fires out if they get started (that is to avoid the kind of perfectionistic thinking that turns lapses into relapses).[22]

Marlatt's view of addictions as overlearned habits is appealing from a self-help perspective. It counters the helplessness experienced by substance abusers in the face of temptation, and it recognizes the need for strategies to prevent lapsing episodes from turning into relapse. However, it would be unfortunate if addicts misinterpreted talk regarding the normalcy of lapsing as an invitation to do so. Furthermore, if, in fact, a certain form of substance abuse—alcoholism in particular—*is* a disease, then addicts may underestimate the biological basis for the abuse and sabotage recovery by persisting at efforts to drink moderately.

It may help us to accept temporary lapses more fully to discover that behaviors once learned and then discontinued can be relearned with only 20 percent of the original effort. Moreover, it is helpful to know that skills once mastered are still valuable *even when not used*. Fear turns into panic when one feels helpless. Knowing that you have the skills to handle the stressor prevents the fear from becoming panic, even if you do not use them.

## Summary

This chapter has been devoted to a review of the basics of change. There is a science and technology of change and mastering those basic principles will turn helplessness into resourcefulness. Such knowledge is empowering. It allows us to approach difficult life situations with confidence. The resulting sense of control prepares us to view demands as challenges rather than as stressors.

Successful change requires careful preparation. We must clearly identify what needs to be changed. To prevent sagging motivation, it is important to recognize and accept the costs of changing before we begin. It also is important to analyze the context in which troublesome behavior occurs. This involves uncovering events that cue and reward the behavior and, where possible, eliminating them. It also involves deciding upon replacement behaviors and attempting to set up a context of cues and consequences in which they are more likely to occur. Attention should be directed to the desired behavior, for one's energy follows one's attention. Rewarding conditions should be set up to reinforce the desired behavioral change. Feedback regarding progress is highly rewarding, and to be effective it requires continuous recording of results.

Change requires adequate motivation, careful planning, and practice over an extended period of time. Efforts to change follow an uneven course. A trend is the proper measure of progress. Ask only "Am I doing better this week than last, this month than last?" Lapsing is normal, and relapsing is to be expected from time to time. Perfectionism is brittle and leads to the collapse of motivation. Fight feelings of guilt over lapsing and relapsing because it only steals energy from your efforts to change. Remind yourself that the more times you try to break old habits and to establish new ones, the more likely you are to succeed.

Controlling one's attention is vital to successful change. Attending to something gives it energy. Focusing on failures or successes makes them more likely. We guide behavior with our attention and imagination. In the next chapter we examine the powerful effects of attention and imagination upon behavior.

**Exhibit 6–3.** Solution to the Nine-dot Problem

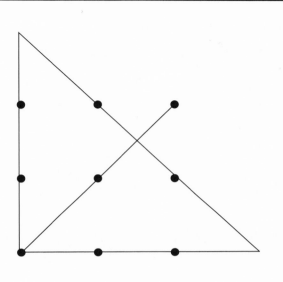

## ENDNOTES

1. Hugh Prather, *Nores to Myself* (Moab, Utah: Real People Press, 1970).

2. Richard Bach, *Jonathan Livingston Seagull* (New York: Macmillan, 1970).

3. James Kavanaugh, *Celebrate the Sun* (Plainview, New York: Dutton, 1973).

4. Archibald MacLeish, "The Great American Frustration," *Saturday Review*, 13 July 1968, 13–16.

5. Jiddu Krishnamurti, *Think on These Things* (New York: Harper and Row, 1970).

6. Eric Fromme, "Values, Psychology, and Human Existence," in *New Knowledge In Human Values*, ed. Abraham Maslow (New York: Harper, 1959).

7. Dan Greenburg, *How to Be a Jewish Mother* (Los Angeles: Price, Stern, Sloan, 1965), 32.

8. Hans Selye, *Stress Without Distress* (New York: New American Library, 1974).

9. Sheldon Kopp, *The Hanged Man: Psychotherapy of the Forces of Darkness* (Palo Alto: Science and Behavior Books, 1974), 6.

10. Ibid., 144.

11. Jean Piaget, *The Psychology of Intelligence* (New York: Harcourt, Brace & World, 1950).

12. William Blake, "The Marriage of Heaven and Hell," in *The Complete Writings of William Blake*, ed. Geoffrey Keynes (New York: New American Library, 1966), 148.

13. Arthur Koestler, *The Sleepwalkers* (New York: Grosset and Dunlap, 1963), 74.

14. Shunryu Suzuki, *Zen Mind, Beginner's Mind* (New York: Weatherhill, 1970).

15. Richard Fisch, J. Weakland, and L. Segal, *Tactics of Change: Doing Things Badly* (San Francisco: Jossey-Bass, 1982).

16. Paul Watzlawick, J. Weakland, and R. Fisch, *Change: Principles of Problem Formation and Problem Resolution* (New York: Norton, 1974).

17. Gary P. Latham and Edwin A. Locke, "Goal Setting—A Motivational Technique That Works," in *Motivation and Work Behavior*, ed. Richard M. Steers and Lyman W. Porter (New York: McGraw-Hill, 1987), 121.

18. Adam Smith, *Powers of Mind* (New York: Random House, 1975).

19. Alan Marlatt, "Relapse Prevention: A Self-Control Program for the Treatment of Addictive Behaviors," in *Adherence, Compliance, and Generalization in Behavioral Medicine*, ed. R. B. Stuart (New York: Brunner/Mazel, 1982).

20. Alan Marlatt and J. R. Gordon, *Relapse Prevention* (New York: Guilford Press, 1985).

21. C. Cummings, J. R. Gordon, and Alan Marlatt, "Relapse: Prevention and Prediction," in *The Addictive Disorders: Treatment of Alcoholism Drug Abuse, Smoking, and Obesity*, ed. W. R. Miller (New York: Pergamon Press, 1980).

22. Kelly D. Brownell, *The LEARN Program for Weight Control* (Philadelphia: University of Pennsylvania Medical Press, 1986).

# CHAPTER SEVEN

# "IMAGINEERING" CHANGE

Imagination is more important than knowledge.
——Albert Einstein

In the province of the mind, what one believes
to be true, either is true or becomes true.
——John Lilly

Much of our behavior is triggered by dominant thoughts and images of ourselves. These self-images serve as prophecies that we earnestly set out to fulfill. We shape our behavior until it becomes a reasonable facsimile of these mental images. These images serve as templates against which behavior is constantly compared. The effort to conform to these images is not totally conscious; indeed, it is quite likely that many of these mental guides are unconscious life-scripts. In a sense all people are actors practicing to portray faithfully these lifescripts. Some of these scripts are for losers; others, for winners. Losers, winners, heroes, villains—whatever the role, much behavior seems calculated to fulfill the prescribed script.

Once we become aware of how these unconscious scripts influence us, we can strengthen our motivation to replace stressful, self-sabotaging habits by the creative use of the imagination. We have called this effort "imagineering" because such creative use of the imagination combines imagery with the actual engineering of change. Changing our estimates of what is possible—learning to see ourselves as capable—can create energy with which to effect personal change.

197

# Sharpening the Picture

Carefully defined goals are more attractive than ambiguous ones. Mark Twain once said, "You can't depend on your eyes when your imagination is out of focus." When the picture of a goal is fuzzy, when the signposts are out-of-focus, it is difficult to maintain a sense of direction and momentum. A clear mental picture of the destination can greatly increase the resolve to persist in the face of the pain that is part of personal growth. In animal psychology there is a phenomenon called goal gradient. Researchers have noted that animals increase their striving for a goal when it comes more clearly in sight. Racing greyhounds, for example, are egged on when a rabbit is close to them. For humans, the sharper the picture of a goal, the greater its magnetism. Consequently, time spent in defining the exact nature of the behavior desired is a step toward improving our motivation.

**In his autobiography** *Second Wind,* Bill Russell—one of the most accomplished athletes of the National Basketball Association—beautifully describes how bringing an image into proper perspective can influence performance. He was selected for the high school basketball team because he was exceptionally tall, even though he was awkward and gangly. He seldom played, however, and because the team had one less uniform than players, he got to wear a uniform only half of the time. While on tour, he had occasion to watch the premier center McKelvey make his turn toward the basket and gracefully dunk the ball. It seemed so natural, so fluid. Again and again he watched the movement with awe. Gradually he saw himself making the same skillful motions with the ball going through the hoop. After mastering the moves in his imagination, he entered the game with surprising results. He wrote:

> When I went into the game, I grabbed an offensive rebound and put it into the basket just the way McKelvey did. It seemed natural, almost as if I were just stepping into a film and following the signs. When the imitation worked and the ball went in, I could hardly contain myself. I was so elated I thought I'd float right out of the gym. Every time I'd tried to copy moves in the past, I'd dribbled the ball off my arm or committed some other goof. Now for the first time, I had transferred something from my head to my body. It seemed so easy.[1]

Too often we resist the work involved in clearly defining our goals and settle instead for ambiguous statements. When the goal is fuzzy, it is difficult both to find the starting gate and to measure progress en route. For example, we may decide to improve our social relationships. Yet, such a vague statement offers little in the way of practical guidance. This general expression of a goal must be translated into a more specific statement that says what improved social relationships means on a personal basis. Are we referring to a need to be more or less assertive with others? To become more spontaneous and less guarded when in the company of others? To develop the skill and courage to express appreciation and affection for others? To become more comfortable in groups? Any or all of these may be involved in a general goal implied in improved social relationships.

In refining a goal statement, we need to be as specific as possible. If by improved social relationships, we hope to increase our comfort in the presence of others, then we should begin to think primarily about an index of comfort in groups. The goal can be made even more specific. Are we referring to comfort experienced as a spectator or as a participant? What kind of group settings are meant? What kind of participation is unsettling? This dogged pursuit of a more meaningful goal statement may result in the translation of an expression as general as "improved social relationships" to one as specific as "less anxiety experienced while presenting views to fellow workers at the office." Although it is not easy to arrive at so detailed a form, the specific nature of the second goal statement is helpful in suggesting a strategy for attacking the problem and in measuring progress. It is indeed difficult to continue a journey when we are not certain where we are going or whether we are closer to, or farther from, the goal than when we began.

As a rule of thumb, we should not settle for a goal statement that does not suggest immediate steps for its accomplishment, along with a reasonably clear basis for measuring progress. Anything less is destructive to motivation for change.

## Anticipating Success

Infrahuman species lack the well-developed associative areas of the human brain. Consequently, they are unable to project themselves in time and space, an ability necessary for imagination. The well-developed human nervous system is endowed with this dubious advantage; it is dubious because the same associative network that enables people to project themselves in time and space also enables them to worry.

This superior endowment also enables us to objectify ourselves, to hold in our minds images or pictures of ourselves. Most behavior is consistent with these self-images. It is still a matter of dispute among psychologists as to whether these self-images are merely an abstract of existing behavior, or whether, once established, they assume independent existences and serve to produce consistency in behavior. Some schools of psychology, namely, the self-theorists or phenomenologists, stress the determinative function of the self-image. We authors tend to agree with this view; that is, once the self-image emerges, it appears to be a major source of influence upon behavior.

Changes in the self-image are reflected in our behavior. An effort to alter self-image has served as the focus of treatment for many therapists. It is well represented in the academic literature by Carl Rogers and George Kelly, and in the popular literature by Maxwell Maltz and others.[2]

A solid realistic self-image is essential to our personal growth and development. When we are comfortable and honest with ourselves about strengths and weaknesses, we are more likely to have the energy and desire to pursue growth. Unfortunately, many of us either hold inappropriately low estimates of our worth, or we hold brittle fantasied versions of ourselves. Either extreme reflects an inadequate self-concept and will limit our functioning. There are many bases for the belief that we should love ourselves: for example, believing that we are made in the image of a loving Creator, that life is a part of the journey to a perfect state, or that man is the fittest of creatures pursuing the mastery of survival. The universal belief, however, is our need to value our identity and existence as an enabling condition for self-actualization.

Thus, negating one's worth is self-defeating. In denying our value, we deny ourselves some critical rights. For example, each of us has the right to an individuality that comprises our assets and liabilities. We also have the right to receive from life all that it offers. In limiting our worth, there is very little possibility of happiness and peace; instead we experience confusion, unrest, and misery. Without appreciating ourselves, we deny ourselves the right to receive the goodnesses of life, and ultimately we have little to offer others. Harvey Milkman and Stanley Sunderwirth reported that a crucial factor in all addictions is low self-regard, and "manifest or masked, it is basic to most dysfunctional lifestyles."[3]

This self-love should also be realistic. Many of us live behind masks to such a degree that our own reflection bears the image of a mask. We cannot accept our limitations and, thus, we deny them. Tragically, this leads us to an accumulation of experiences that we refuse to accept. To honestly recognize our limitations is not debilitating. Rather, when we allow ourselves to love the fullness of our humanity, both good and bad, our weaknesses serve as links in the chain that connects us to our fellow man and become the catalysts of change and growth. When we can appreciate our limitations in this light, we can abandon our shallow painted walls and enter the rich landscape of human experience.

The desire for self-change assumes that we value our lives enough to seek the very best for them. If we fail to meet this initial requirement, then our first priority is to examine our core self-image and work to develop genuine self-love. Without this, any personal fine tuning merely leaves us spinning our wheels and going nowhere. We will not grasp any personal satisfaction from self-change without self-esteem. Self-esteem is a basic need we must attend to first.

How do we come to see ourselves differently? And how do we accept new images of ourselves so completely that they affect our behavior? Some therapists believe that such images cannot be changed by a frontal attack. They believe that the self-image is the product of interaction with significant others, that we accept a view of ourselves that we see reflected in the eyes of others. The self-image, therefore, would represent a perception of the way others see us. According to this view, we must have help from others to change our self-images. Therapy consists of a corrective emotional experience wherein we come to accept troublesome aspects of ourselves more fully. Because we prize the opinion of the therapist, his or her acceptance of these troublesome behaviors serves as a direct rebuttal to what we previously perceived to be the negative responses of others; and, thus, in due time the self-image is altered in a more realistic direction.

## Frontal Attacks on the Self-image

Other therapists maintain that a frontal attack on self-image is most effective. They argue as follows: if we change the words we use to describe ourselves to ourselves, and if we practice holding different pictures of ourselves, then we can, in time, effectively improve the self-image. The trick, these therapists say, is to perceive ourselves as already having made the change.

Maltz's theory, called psychocybernetics, advocates direct attack upon inadequate self-images. His theory comes from *cybernetics*, a Greek word meaning "steersmanship," and *psyche*, another Greek word meaning "mind." The title fits Maltz's position well since his views stress the purposiveness of human nature. Humans are not divided into two warring minds. Maltz does not view the conscious and unconscious minds as being antagonistic. Rather, they work cooperatively, with the conscious mind being responsible for goal setting. The conscious mind has a servant responsible for furnishing the means and muscles for accomplishing goals. This servant which others have called the Unconscious, is called by Maltz the Automatic Mechanism.[4]

The Automatic Mechanism does not have a mind of its own. It is the willing servant of the conscious mind; it is a slave that seeks quietly and covertly to carry out the will of the mind. It works like a servomechanism, an automatic guidance system. It may be programmed by the mind for success or failure. If it is fed information to the effect that we are unworthy, inferior, undeserving, or incapable, then it will guide our behaviors accordingly. Conversely, if we feed it information based on a positive self-image, it will order up behavior compatible with such an image. Thus, we create ourselves out of the goals and images we feed into our Automatic Mechanism. If we feed it success goals, it will function as a Success Mechanism; if we feed it negative goals, it will function as a Failure Mechanism.

The trick then is to achieve a self-image that is positive and enhancing. But the self-image is a product of experiences. Are we not, therefore, condemned to live out our days enslaved by a self-image that reflects our past experiences? The answer lies in a deeper understanding of the manner in which the human nervous system functions. It cannot tell the difference between real and synthetic experiences. Experiences that are imagined are as much the cement and bricks of a self-image as those that are real.

It is, after all, not actual experiences that affect us, but rather our interpretation of these experiences. An early Roman philosopher, Epictetus (60 A.D.), once said, "Men are disturbed not by things, but by the view which they take of them. When we meet with troubles, become anxious or depressed, let us never blame anyone but . . . our opinions about things."[5] Several centuries later William James concluded, "since you make them [facts] evil or good by your own thoughts about them, it is the ruling of your thoughts which proves to be your principal concern."[6]

We never know exactly what the facts are in any situation. Indeed, in any one day there are facts that can justify either a pessimistic or an optimistic view of ourselves. The good perceptions are as genuine as are the evil ones. Our perceptions are not a matter of intellectual honesty or dishonesty; they are merely a matter of what we choose to focus upon.

Focus upon the negative, and we turn our Automatic Mechanism into a Failure Mechanism; focus upon the positive and we turn it into a Success Mechanism. Further, if we are unhappy with our mental images, then we can change them by creatively picturing ourselves differently and by acting as if this new picture is an accurate representation.

Getting a clear fix on the nature of a solution takes us a long way toward successful problem solving. The first order of the day in self-change strategies, then, is to fashion a clear mental picture of ourselves as we would be if we had already changed. The second order is to hold such an image steadfastly in mind. Attention is either a powerful ally or a powerful enemy. If it focuses upon failure, then failure it is likely to be; if it focuses upon success, then we are much more likely to be successful. How can we, then, constantly attend to successful self-images if we are programmed to think of ourselves as failures?

The attention span of the human mind is brief. It jumps rapidly from one thing to another. For this reason, we will be able to center attention for a longer time upon successful self-images if we embellish them with vivid details. If we are attempting to lose weight, for example, we must mentally picture ourselves as slim and trim. We might imagine our svelte figure reflected nude in a full-length mirror. We might focus upon a midsection taut with well-developed muscles and totally devoid of the usual doughnut of fat. Perhaps we can imagine the envious response of friends and acquaintances, who admiringly notice our willowy form on the beach or at the community pool. Not only can we *see* the slender form, but we can *feel* the extra surge of energy freed by the loss of excessive, ugly fat. We feel ourselves effortlessly getting up out of a deep-cushioned chair and sprightfully walking off. Perhaps we focus attention on how our clothes will look when we are slim. Perhaps we see ourselves entering the office of a local seamstress and proudly requesting that the seams be taken in several inches, or perhaps we decide that our new images will now allow us to choose more modern styles — or perhaps we are now entitled to consider replacing the old wardrobe with one containing some of the styles we have admired on others.

If our goal is to become more comfortable in the view we present to colleagues, then once again we must engage our creative imagination to paint in vivid detail a picture of ourselves as we confidently express ourselves at work. We sense the calm mental state that can expel the usually feverish condition of fear and anxiety. We hear ourselves speaking slowly and articulately in a voice that is rhythmical and firm. We are poised and content to express our views without necessarily persuading others of them. There is no trace in our voice of the used-car salesman's pitch. We recognize that it is not overly important that others agree, or that we agree with them for that matter. But we sense that what we have to say will be of interest to them. We see ourselves accurately expressing views, and we see others looking at one another and nodding agreement or otherwise indicating interest in our opinions.

It is important to spend time creating and rehearsing our goals. We must have these mental experiences repeatedly, and having them means experiencing them in detail. If we are having difficulty with the creation of such themes or mental pictures, we can ask for the assistance of trusted companions, who can often add considerably to versions of our imagined goals. They can dip into their own experiences and greatly embellish the pictures. We can also prod the imagination with models furnished by acquaintances, films, or books. By selecting the sources upon which we wish to focus, we modify our self-image, and by modifying our self-image, we modify behavior.

These products of creative imaginations furnish guidelines for new roles to be acted out. Again, we begin to *act as if* these new self-images are real. The new role or life-script may seem artificial and unnatural at first, and we may even feel hypocritical. We may conclude that we are acting out of character—that this new behavior is false. The new behavior at first is unnatural; it is unreal, and indeed, *this is precisely why we are performing the behavior.* After all, we have decided that we want to change, and changing involves changing behavior. Present habits that now feel so natural were also learned. We are not born with habits. Undoubtedly present habits felt just as artificial when we were first experimenting with them as these new behaviors now feel. If we persist in role-playing long enough, we will find that the new behaviors eventually become habits, and it will no longer be necessary to play a role.

Since we have little understanding of the extensive amount of time it takes to master present roles, we are apt to become impatient while trying out new roles. We hesitatingly begin to practice a new life-script and soon despair of the possibility that we will ever be able to "act that way." Our efforts are foredoomed to failure because the lack of faith precludes us from being able to play the roles with abandonment. Such feelings can persist in the face of very slow change.

Self-change is a slow process—even when the formula for change is exquisitely appropriate. Maltz suggested that it usually takes about twenty-one days to effect any perceptible change in a self-image. He reminds us that it takes about twenty-one days for patients of plastic surgery to get used to their new faces, about the same amount of time for the phantom limb to disappear from the mind of an amputee, and about the same time for a new house to seem comfortable.

We must go on practicing a new image for some time without seeing the results. This is parallel to a concept in physics called critical mass: physicists point out that energy must often amass over a period of time before it perceptibly changes form. For example, we can heat water for quite a while before it changes into steam. Its temperature may reach 100 degrees, 150 degrees, or even 200 degrees Fahrenheit without any visible evidence that change is occurring. Only after water reaches critical mass at 211 degrees does it miraculously change its form from liquid to gas. The process of self-change is very much the same. Early efforts often seem unrewarding; we seem to be using a frightful lot of energy and willpower for no perceptible reward. Approaching critical mass is not very reinforcing. Motivation is greatly strengthened, however, when we begin to reach critical mass.

If we persist in the tedious work of self-change, then we must come to believe in the importance of the repetitive efforts involved in approaching critical mass. We must continue to practice the role, to imagine ourselves as we would like to be, even when behavior stubbornly refuses to go along.

A new self-image must be a reasonable facsimile of our present self. It must roughly correspond to reality. We could imagine ourselves able to fly without wings, or as Jesus Christ or Napoleon Bonaparte, but such images have an obvious air of unreality. An image must be a reasonable facsimile of a self we honestly believe we can become.

Early efforts to change an image often employ a process behavioral psychologists call shaping. Shaping refers to efforts to reward improvement. We do not expect full-blown, perfect performance—we only expect a reasonable approximation of it. Once we have approached this level of performance, we can raise the bar of the hurdle a bit higher. Any attempt at self-change involves rounds of approximations, tedious effort, and self-endorsement. Another format used in attempts to change the self image is autosuggestive techniques.

# Autosuggestive Techniques

Autosuggestive techniques have been used informally for centuries and formally for many decades to increase human motivation. The techniques are related to hypnosis; indeed, the practice of autosuggestion is sometimes called autohypnosis. Both require a highly relaxed, unstimulated state.

Throughout the ages, hypnotic-like states have been used by healers. There were the sleep temples in Greece and Egypt, where priests used forms of hypnosis to treat physical ailments. Trance induction is frequently brought on in primitive cultures through drums, dancing, and chanting.

The eighteenth-century Frenchman Anton Mesmer combined the use of trance-like states with his metaphysical views of astrology to form a unique treatment of physical problems. He believed that the human body was analogous to a magnet, with the top and bottom halves emitting opposite attractions. He thought diseases were caused by an imbalance in the magnetic poles of the body and could be cured by restoring the magnetic balance. His method was to pass magnetic rods over the bodies of patients until they were persuaded that the previously interrupted universal flow of magnetism was restored to its natural rhythm. Mesmer had begun to recognize the significance of suggestion and persuasion in the therapeutic process.

An Englishman, James Braid, coined the term *hypnosis* from the Greek word for sleep, *hypnos.* He dropped the metaphysical trappings of Mesmer's system and induced trances via eye fixations. The applications of hypnosis spread rapidly to the medical field. The center of the use of hypnosis in medicine moved to the Nancy Clinic in France, where Freud was to become interested in the technique under the mentorship of Charcot.

A French druggist, Emile Coue, also studied at the Nancy Clinic. He later abandoned the use of the trance and began the practice of "waking suggestion"—autosuggestion. He is said to have discovered this to be more effective than drugs. The flavor of his method can be savored in the following excerpt from his manual:

> Therefore, every time you have a pain, physical or otherwise, you will go quietly to your room . . . sit down and shut your eyes, pass your hand lightly across your forehead if it is mental distress, or upon the part that hurts, if it is pain in any part of the body, repeat the words: "It is going, it is going," etc. very rapidly, even at the risk of babbling . . . . The essential idea is to say: "It is going, it is

going" so quickly that it is impossible for a thought of contrary nature to force itself between the words. We thus actually think it is going, and as all ideas that we fix upon the mind become a reality to us, the pain, physical or mental, vanishes.[7]

Coue abandoned the trance induction entirely, insisting that all suggestion is in reality nothing but autosuggestion.

The British Medical Association officially endorsed hypnosis in 1955 and the American Medical Association followed in 1958. The method is used primarily by psychiatrists in an effort to integrate psychodynamic material more effectively. Specific hypnotic techniques have been developed for age regression, scene visualization, imagery activity, fantasy evocation, hypnography, and other modifications of perceptual functions.

The current trend is toward an emphasis on a person's conscious cooperation and away from an inactive and passive posture. In this sense, Coue's preference for waking suggestion appears to have gained support. Theodore Barber, a leading researcher in hypnosis, has concluded, as did Coue, that the trance is not necessary to hypnosis, that hypnosis is a matter of conscious expectancy.[8] Jerome Frank, in *Persuasion and Healing*, pointed out that the faith healer, witch doctor, shaman, medicine man, and psychotherapists alike all manage to help a demoralized patient by raising expectations.[9]

If, then, the conscious expectancy can be manipulated by persuasion and suggestion, behavior appropriate to the expectancy will follow. Practitioners of autosuggestion maintain that such persuasion and suggestion can come from ourselves — that we can engineer our own behavior through this technique.

The Russian psychologist, Platonov, maintains that there is a close connection between mental activity and the physical processes that may be responsive to suggestions. He believes that all symbolic images evoke some type of physiological response. He quotes Pavlov, who formulated the following principle:

> As long as you think of a certain movement (that is, you have a kinesthetic idea) you involuntarily perform it without noticing it. Thus, each time we think of a movement, we actually perform it abortively.[10]

It follows from this principle that mental practice of a performance may smooth out the actual performance itself. There is some research evidence to suggest that such athletic performances as dart throwing and basketball shooting may be improved by daily mental practice.[11] We might facetiously speculate that Professor Harold Hill in the Broadway production *The Music Man* may not have been totally without justification when he frantically urged his Iowa school children to "think music."

In order to prepare yourself for the maximum benefits from autosuggestion, the body should be placed in a state of quiescence and passivity. Find a comfortable posture—usually a sitting or reclining position is best. Begin a set of relaxation exercises in which you alternately tense and relax each part of the body. A muscle relaxes more easily if it is first tensed. A suggested order for this is hands, arms, forehead, eyes, mouth, tongue, neck, shoulders, stomach, buttocks, thighs, calves, feet and toes. Tense the muscle, hold it for five to seven seconds, relax it, and then repeat the exercise. While the pattern may take twenty to thirty minutes at first, you will eventually be able to short-circuit it by combining muscle groups.

After the body feels relaxed, begin counting from ten to one, taking a deep breath for each number. When the count is completed, follow with a key word, such as "relax." If the relaxation exercises are followed enough times by the counting and the word "relax," you will soon be able to induce a similarly relaxed state merely by counting and repeating the word "relax."

Some people find it helpful to focus on an imaginary object, such as a spot in the middle of the eyebrows, to suppress other thoughts that might interfere with their concentration. Once the routine for relaxation has been mastered, the state may be achieved within a few minutes under most circumstances.

With the body and mind stilled, you can begin making self-suggestions. Sontged recommended four rules for enhancing the effects of self-suggestion:

1. *Make suggestions positive and permissive.* Most people assume a resistive stance when pressed or coerced; therefore a permissive suggestion such as "I can . . . " is more likely to be carried out than a more domineering one such as "I will . . ."
2. *Repeat suggestions to increase their strength.* Suggestions should be repeated three or four times during a single session. This principle of repetition is well-respected in the advertising world. People tend to believe an idea if they hear it often enough.
3. *Phrase suggestions in the present perfect rather than in the*

*present tense*. The Unconscious (Automatic Mechanism) needs time to act on suggestions. Rather than saying, "My headache is gone," it is more effective to say "My headache is beginning to clear up." Such a statement is more believable in this form, and it is only when we come to believe a suggestion that it is acted upon by the unconscious.

4. *Employ visual images in suggestions whenever possible*. Imagine yourself subjectively experiencing the desired goal rather than objectively observing the activity.[12]

These techniques are designed to influence a basic part of our personality mentioned before called the Unconscious, or the Automatic Mechanism. Most people are living out unconscious scripts that can lead either to success or failure. People write their own scripts containing their own positive or negative goals and self-images. These techniques call for a frontal assault on inadequate and negative self-thoughts and feelings. If we persist at attending to specific, positive goals, rather than allowing our minds to fret fearfully over the possibility of failure; if we construct new, synthetic experiences to replace the old, hurtful ones by creatively imagining them vividly and in detail; if we properly prepare our minds and bodies by relaxation for positive autosuggestions—if we do these things consistently and persistently over time—we may expect our motivation for self-improvement to increase and our lifestyles to change in positive directions.

## ENDNOTES

1. Bill Russell and Taylor Branch, *Second Wind: The Memoirs of an Opinionated Man* (New York: Simon and Schuster, 1979), 67.

2. Carl Rogers, *Client-Centered Therapy* (Boston: Houghton Mifflin, 1951); George A. Kelly, *Theory of Personality: The Psychology of Personal Constructs* (New York: Norton, 1963); Maxwell Maltz, *Psycho-Cybernetics* (Hollywood, CA: Wilshire, 1960).

3. Harvey Milkman and Stanley Sunderwirth, "Craving for Ecstasy," *Psychology Today* (October 1983): 36–44.

4. Maltz, *Psycho-Cybernetics*.

5. Epictetus in *The New Guide to Rational Living*, ed. Albert Ellis and Robert A. Harper (North Hollywood, California: Wilshire, 1976).

6. William James, *Principles of Psychology, II* (New York: Dover, 1890).

7. Emile Coue, *How To Practice Suggestion and Autosuggestion* (New York: American Library Service, 1923), 43.

8. Theodore Barber, N. Spanos, and W. DeMoor, "Hypnosis and Behavior Therapy: Common Denominators," *American Journal of Clinical Hypnosis* 16 (1973): 45–62.

9. Jerome Frank, *Persuasion and Healing* (New York: Schocken, 1975).

10. K. K. Platonov, "Method of Verbal Suggestion," in *Active Psychotherapy,* ed. Harold Greenwald (Atherton Press, 1967), 234.

11. Richard Suinn, "Body Thinking: Psychology for Olympic Champs," *Psychology Today* (July 1976): 38–43.

12. A. Sontged, *Self-Hypnosis*, Automated Learning, Inc., 1972. Audio-tape.

# CHAPTER EIGHT

# SEEKING OUTSIDE HELP

Bad company is loss, and good company is gain: . . .
In company with the wind the dust flies heaven-ward;
if it joins water, it becomes mud and sinks.
——Tulsi Das

How many a man has dated a new era in his life
from the reading of a book.
——Thoreaux

Reading is to the mind what exercise is to the body.
——Richard Steele

Thus far, this volume has emphasized the helping of oneself and others to overcome stress and helplessness though one's own efforts. We have discussed the interrelatedness of all of us and the seeming dilemma of being independent and yet dependent. However, we have also emphasized the resources individuals can muster internally with the proper mind-sets and the use of a cadre of psychotechnical aids. We hope that in our hyperbolic bias toward the use of one's own internal resources we have not misled the reader to believe that there is no help out *there.* This chapter points to outside help in the form of groups that specialize in adjustment problems, trained professionals who treat stress, and finally, books that are often prescribed for some of the distresses of life.

## Choosing Our Company

Group pressure is a powerful influence on behavior. We are often dragged down from our lofty resolutions by the company of people who do not share our goals. On the other hand, we are sometimes motivated to pursue nobler ends by the good examples of others. If we wish to strengthen our motivation to change, then we obviously should choose our company wisely.

When we attempt to break old habits and form new ones, we should seek the company of others who will serve as appropriate models. Having firmly established the new behavior, we then may be able successfully to resist negative group influences. It is foolhardy, however, to subject ourselves to unsympathetic audiences before the budding behavior has been adequately rooted. The group's disinterest, or perhaps scorn, for a pursuit may strangle the early growth of improved habits.

Alvin Toffler, in his book *Future Shock*, foresaw the coming self-help group explosion when he recommended "situational grouping" as a strategy for dealing with adjustment problems occasioned by the ever-increasing rate of change in modern society. He quotes Gerjuoy who recommended that temporary groups be formed for "families caught in the upheaval of relocation, for men and women about to be divorced, for people about to lose a parent or a spouse, for those about to gain a child, for men preparing to switch to a new occupation, for families that have just moved into a community, for those about to marry off their last child, for those facing retirement—for anyone, in other words, who faces an important life change."[1]

Social psychology devotes much attention to the influence of groups on behavior. The behavior of groups important to individuals has a powerful impact on their behavior. The influence of street gangs upon the behavior of susceptible youth is all too well known to law enforcement personnel. These gangs often prescribe antisocial behaviors and proscribe snitching and other forms of cooperation with the authorities. Reference groups offer identification, support, and a feeling of importance to their members. The socializing influence of religious societies and civic groups upon members is widely believed to be uplifting and positive.

We are social animals, and we depend heavily upon one another for support and guidance. There is a strong tendency to mimic the behavior of significant others. This imitative learning accounts for a significant amount of our behavior, and, consequently, we are well advised to expose ourselves to good behavioral models. A Sufi mystic aptly expressed the idea: "If you don't have room in your living room for an elephant, don't make friends with the elephant trainer."

The reader may be well aware of the fact that existing relationships may sometimes counter the desirable influence of groups we purposefully seek out. The powerful influences of family members, friends, and acquaintances may furnish stiff competition to the selected influences of self-help groups. Exhibit 8–1 depicts these countering influences.

For example, the influence of Weight Watchers meetings in strengthening our resolve to address a weight problem may be countered by the barbs of family members who are threatened by our efforts to attain a healthier, more attractive appearance; or by mothers who take offense at the insinuation that their cooking is a hazard to our health; or a significant other may actually be dependent on our maintaining the behavior or condition we want to change. The increasing number of co-dependency groups gives vivid testimony to this latter phenomenon.

This problem is not easily resolved as it is improbable that we will be able to significantly impact the broader circle of family, friends, and acquaintances in such a way as to cause them to encourage the desired change in our behavior. In more fortunate cases this broader circle may actually support the intended change. Exhibit 8–2 depicts this happy circumstance.

In these cases the broader circle works *with* rather than *against* the

**Exhibit 8–1.** Group Influences That Militate Against One Another

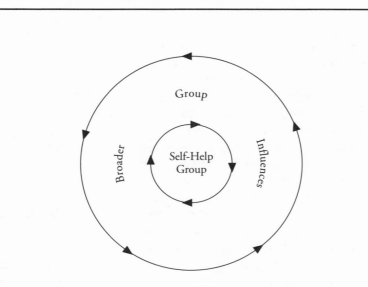

**Exhibit 8–2.** Supportive System Influences

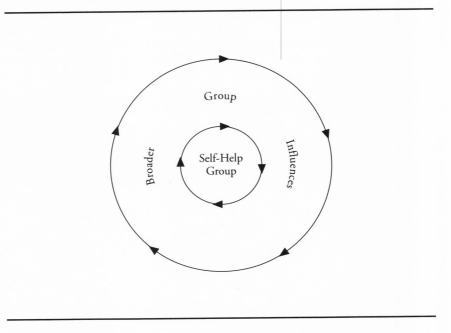

smaller, self-selected group influence. The self-help group becomes a dynamic energizer for change, and its influence, in turn, is further empowered by the broader circle of caring others who want the best for us. In these cases where the broader circle is basically nurturant, we can mobilize its encouragement of our change by carefully apprising it of our intended change in behavior and its importance to us. In any case, whether the broader circle is nurturing or resistive of our desired change, we are helping our cause by purposefully exposing ourselves to the encouraging influences of selected self-help groups.

Self-reliance does not preclude the option of finding others to further our personal goals. We are all influenced by others. Short of a hermetical existence, we cannot escape these group influences. In this chapter we again recommend a self-determining posture, that is, choosing the group influences that we want to impact our behavior. Indeed, some researchers are reporting an increased activity on the part of counselors in connecting individual clients with a wide variety of groups, including self-help groups.[2]

Fortunately, there exist in many communities a number of self-help groups formed to encourage members to change in desirable ways. It may surprise the reader to know that there are approximately one-half million self-help groups in the United States, with memberships of more than fifteen million. Their appeal is unquestionable, and their purposes are as vast as their membership. They may be designed to help members lose weight, stop smoking, avoid alcohol or other drugs, stop gambling or child abuse, study more effectively, exercise, or gain political power. These nonprofessional self-help groups are open to the public. The costs are usually minimal or nonexistent, and members are often self-referred. Many of these groups are extremely helpful to people wishing to make personal changes in their lives. Self-help groups likely will continue their massive growth and become standard practice in struggling with human problems. There are a number of referral sources that can be consulted for assistance in locating an appropriate lay group.

Some states—Georgia, South Dakota, and North Carolina, for example— provide a referral service that offers access to available services throughout the entire state. As an example of how these work, callers in Georgia may dial the tie-line number, indicate the nature of a problem, and receive guidance as to the availability of assistance in their local communities. Referral consultants who handle incoming calls are trained to cut through the usual red tape in an effort to provide an immediate link-up between the consumer and the service agency. Under special conditions, a three-way conversation may take place between the consumer, the referral consultant, and a representative of the service agency.

Other agencies offer services similar to those provided by the state-wide referral agencies, but referrals are limited to a geographical area. The number of a community referral agency can be obtained by telephoning the information number listed under city government or the local United Way. One can often obtain expert referral assistance from a local branch of the National Association for Mental Health, which is a nationwide organization of citizens and consumers of mental health services; consequently, it is likely to be less biased in its referrals than would be the case if it were run by professionals. It is the business of this organization to know what is available publicly and privately. Some local branches also publish directories of community resources that may also list self-help or support groups. One can usually locate the branch number under the listing "Mental Health Association of . . . " in a telephone directory. One of the more accessible referral sources is the

Yellow Pages. In most communities services are listed under the heading "Social Services Organizations."

# Lay Self-help Groups

Many people use the terms *self-help* group and *support* group interchangeably. In practice there is often a subtle distinction—implied by the very difference in terms—between the two groups. The origin of self-help groups in the United States was set in the massive immigrant populations of the early 1900s. Even though social workers sometimes instigated the groups, the groups became popular primarily under lay leadership. In fact, most early self-help groups were suspicious of, if not openly hostile toward, traditional social and psychological treatment methods and programs.

Support groups, on the other hand, are frequently initiated by social agencies and health professionals. Cancer, diabetes, and endometriosis support groups, for example, rely heavily on medical and psychological personnel to consult, provide information, and frequently lead their local groups.

A few of the more important national self-help groups are described in the following pages. Each group's purpose, clientele, frequency of group contact, nature of interaction, fees, and suggested ways of contacting the group are included. The Self-Help Clearing House in Brooklyn, New York, maintains current information on all groups coming to their attention. Any inquiry can be directed to (718) 596–6000.

## Weight Regulation Groups

Losing weight is a difficult task for more than forty million overweight Americans. More difficult still is *keeping weight off* once it is lost. Roughly 80 percent of those who lose weight gain it back during the following year. The need for social support in overcoming health problems such as overweight is great. While some people with iron wills apparently can accomplish the task by themselves, many people strongly need the support of others. In addition, while most people are bored with an overeater's report of indulgence or denial, fellow sufferers may provide the support necessary to persist in fighting this battle. Two of the more successful self-help groups concerned with weight reduction are Weight Watchers and Overeaters Anonymous. One or both are likely to be found in any community.

**Weight Watchers**. The best known of these groups is Weight Watchers. This international organization that has helped millions of people was founded by Jean Nidetch in her home when she sought the help of overweight friends in her efforts to diet.[3] The purpose of the group is to offer support and encouragement for people seeking to lose weight or to maintain previous weight losses. About twenty-five thousand weekly meetings are scheduled in twenty-four countries; seventeen thousand of them are held in the United States. The organization distributes a monthly publication, *Weight Watchers Magazine*, and many supplementary dietary booklets.

Clientele include seriously overweight people, mildly overweight people having difficulty in further trimming, and people wishing to maintain previous weight loss. Weekly meetings begin with a weigh-in. Members mix socially until all are weighed. Each member's weight is publicly announced, provided the weight represents a loss or a weight-loss maintenance. Each victory is applauded. The director leads a discussion of a weight-related topic, and low-calorie recipes are shared. New members are weighed, assigned a goal according to ideal weight tables, and oriented to a diet plan.

After members lose the first 10 pounds, they are rewarded with a pin and given an opportunity to testify before other members about the usefulness of the diet plan. Diet adjustments are made at each 10-pound weight loss and diets are shifted to a special leveling plan when the member is within 10 pounds of the ideal weight. Upon attaining the assigned goal, the member switches to the maintenance plan.

While the diet is useful, the magic of the program seems to lie in the built-in social reinforcement. There is heavy group pressure for weight loss and weekly accountability. The weekly recognition of weight loss is a powerful aid to motivation. The initial registration fee is $25, and a weekly fee ranging from $7 to $10 is collected at each session. A reader may contact the local chapter by consulting the local telephone directory or by writing national headquarters at Weight Watchers, International, Jericho Atrium, 500 N. Broadway, Jericho, NY 11753–2196.

**Overeaters Anonymous.** Overeaters Anonymous is an international organization designed to help compulsive overeaters. It began in the 1960s and patterned itself after the successful Alcoholics Anonymous (AA) program. It has basically adapted the Twelve Step Program of Recovery of AA. While the reader will have a much better idea of the Overeaters Anonymous program after reading the more detailed treatment given AA later in the chapter, a brief description here may be helpful.

The weekly meeting is led by a volunteer leader, who may share a personal experience with the group. The format of the meeting usually calls for discussion, a panel of speakers, or group sharing of experiences. Unlike Weight Watchers, Overeaters Anonymous does not concern itself with food, menus, eating hints, or weighing-in. Like AA, it rests largely on personal testimonies and social support and seeks to get at the basic causes for compulsive eating.

Members are urged to attend meetings several times a week, if possible, and to be honest, open-minded, and willing to help others. There are no fees, but free-will offerings are taken. Consult a local telephone directory for a phone number.

## Addiction-Control Groups

**Alcoholics Anonymous.** Certainly the best known of the self-help groups is Alcoholics Anonymous. More than 76,000 AA groups hold regular weekly meetings worldwide. The World Health Organization called it "the greatest therapeutic organization in the world."[4] This international organization, founded in the 1930s, has assisted thousands of people to live sober, responsible lives. Alcoholics Anonymous often works where doctors, psychiatrists, psychologists, friends, and relatives fail. One reason for its success is the generous social reinforcement afforded members by fellow sufferers. The purpose of the organization is aptly stated in its preamble:

> Alcoholics Anonymous is a fellowship of men and women who share their experience, strength, and hope with each other that they may solve their common problem and help others to recover from alcoholism.
> The only requirement for membership is a desire to stop drinking. There are no dues or fees for AA membership; we are self-supporting through our own contributions.
> AA is not allied with any sect, denomination, political organization, or institution; does not wish to engage in any controversy; neither endorses nor opposes any causes. Our primary purpose is to stay sober and help other alcoholics to achieve sobriety.[5]

The clientele of AA represents a cross-section of Americans. Alcoholism is a common problem, and for that reason one finds in any local association a mixed group of people, representing all professions and varying lifestyles. The organization has a definite religious flavor, although it is not affiliated with any particular religious faith. The religious emphasis is reflected in its Twelve Step Program of Recovery (next page).

## Alcoholics Anonymous Twelve Step Program

1. We admitted we were powerless over alcohol—that our lives had become unmanageable.

2. Came to believe that a Power greater than ourselves could restore us to sanity.

3. Made a decision to turn our will and our lives over to the care of God as we understood Him.

4. Made a searching and fearless moral inventory of ourselves.

5. Admitted to God, to ourselves and to another human being the exact nature of our wrongs.

6. Were entirely ready to have God remove all these defects of character.

7. Humbly asked Him to remove our shortcomings.

8. Made a list of all persons we had harmed, and became willing to make amends to them all.

9. Made direct amends to such people wherever possible, except when to do so would injure them or others.

10. Continued to take personal inventory, and when we were wrong, promptly admitted it.

11. Sought through prayer and meditation to improve our conscious contact with God, as we understood Him, praying only for knowledge of His will for us and the power to carry that out.

12. Having had a spiritual awakening as the result of these steps, we tried to carry this message to alcoholics, and to practice these principles in all our affairs.

There are open and closed AA meetings. In a typical meeting, one is likely to hear the preamble read as well as some encouraging thoughts. The meeting usually includes several personal testimonials by members. These are generally nondefensive, poignant accounts of past bouts with drinking or present attempts to resist. The atmosphere is warm and supportive.

New members are urged to attend meetings every night for 90 days. Thereafter, it is customary to attend at least one meeting per week, but many members regularly attend two, three, or four meetings per week. Members are expected to help others seeking to break the habit at whatever the hour of the day or night. Members often testify during meetings of their trips across town to hold the hand of new members throughout the night as they try to kick the habit. Certainly this effort and the social reinforcement provided in the meetings contribute largely to the phenomenal success of AA. Contact may be made with representatives through the local telephone directory or by writing to the national headquarters at P.O. Box 459, Grand Central Station, New York, NY 10163. Telephone: (212) 686–1100.

Alcoholics Anonymous' Alateen Family Groups also exist for those concerned about someone else's drinking problem. Groups for adult children of alcoholics are also widely available.

**Gamblers Anonymous.** Gamblers Anonymous is an international organization formed to help compulsive gamblers stop gambling. Gambling is as much an obsession for some people as alcohol is for others. One member disclosed to the writers that he flew from Atlanta to Miami six times during one week to attend horse races. Many gamblers find that an association with others who share their problem is crucial to their recovery.

As the name would indicate, Gamblers Anonymous is patterned after Alcoholics Anonymous. The meetings follow the AA format — public confession and group support. The group practices twelve steps to recovery, which are similar to those of Alcoholics Anonymous. There appear to be three main ingredients of the program: (1) recognizing that one is powerless to break the habit, (2) dependence upon the mutual aid of the association, and (3) missionary work to help other gamblers to break the habit. Again the interest and support of others are very important to this group, as they are to most other self-help groups.

New members are urged to attend meetings nightly, if possible, In some communities in New York, New Jersey, and California, this is possible due to the large number of local chapters. The organization is growing rapidly, and there is even Gam-Anon for spouses of gamblers.

There are no fees, but free-will offerings are taken. Representatives can be contacted through the local telephone directory in most large cities. National offices are located at P.O. Box 17173, Los Angeles, CA 90017. Telephone: (213) 386–8789.

**Cocaine Anonymous.** Cocaine Anonymous has a network of about one thousand chapters in the United States and Canada, but members sometimes will go to any "Twelve Step Program". All "Anonymous" groups have in common the twelve-point statement of beliefs acknowledging the members' need for help. Information on Cocaine Anonymous can be obtained from Cocaine Anonymous Worldwide Services Office, P.O. Box 1367, Culver City, CA 90239. Telephone: (213) 559–5833.

**Smokers' Groups.** Many communities have Smokers Anonymous groups listed in the local newspaper. Also, some chapters of the American Lung Association sponsor smoking-withdrawal workshops. One such group meets for five consecutive evenings. A leader recites the dangers involved in the habit and presents techniques for breaking the habit. A buddy system is used. The leader also makes telephone contact with members each day of the workshop. The fee, a modest $10, is charged to encourage attendance. Once again, social reinforcement seems to be the prime motivation. Contact the local chapter of the American Lung Association in any community or 1–800–4CANCER for information regarding the existences of similar programs.

There are a growing number of commercial programs for smoking withdrawal. Since they are profit-making organizations, the expense involved is sometimes large. Smoke Enders has numerous offices in the United States and Canada. It charges $175 for a nine-week program. The weekly meetings last for two hours. This program is based upon many of the behavior principles covered in chapter 4. The address for the national office is Smoke Enders, Phillipsburg, NJ 08865.

## Emotional Control Groups

Some self-help groups are concerned with helping members to better manage their emotions. Most of us have suffered the tyranny of runaway emotions at times, but some people contend with more serious emotional disturbances. Recovery, Inc. and Emotions Anonymous are well-known groups for people with serious emotional problems.

**Recovery, Inc.** This is an international self-help group begun in Chicago in 1937 by Abraham A. Low, M.D. It has about ten thousand members in 1,025 chapters representing all fifty states as well as Canada and Puerto Rico.[6] It offers former mental patients a systematic method of self-help aftercare and assists other people who consider themselves to be chronically nervous. Approximately half the members have never been hospitalized for mental illness, and 30 percent have never been treated for an emotional condition.[7] The range of members extends from people with nervous symptoms, including depression, anxiety attacks, racing thoughts, sleeplessness, suicidal thoughts, fatigue, and hopelessness to mental patients who at one time were hospitalized. However, openly disturbed people are never invited to meetings, which are held weekly. The Recovery method consists of (1) independent study of Low's book, *Mental Health Through Will Training* and other publications by him;[8] (2) regular attendance at the weekly meetings; and (3) the practice of Recovery principles in daily life.

Meetings are open to the public and are led by a Recovery-trained volunteer. Mental health professionals cannot become leaders. Leaders are lay people pursuing the Recovery method for their own emotional health. They have had training in the method at the Recovery training site and receive ongoing training throughout the year.

The meetings are quite structured. They begin with listening to one of Dr. Low's records or a reading from his book. Volunteers then offer recent examples of experiences that they have attempted to handle by the Recovery principles. These examples are presented in four structured steps described by Dr. Low. Each person is limited to 5 minutes; then 10 minutes are allotted to discussion of the example by remaining members. Each meeting lasts approximately 1 hour.

A brief social may follow the formal meeting. The conversation is expected to center on Recovery principles as they can be applied to daily living. Members may contact one another by telephone for aid at other times, but must limit the call to 5 minutes.

Recovery, Inc. is nonsectarian, is not intended to supplant the psychiatrist, doctor, or other mental health professional, and does not offer diagnosis or individual counseling. It merely attempts to apply the Recovery principles to those aspects of the person's life that allow for self-guidance. One member summed up his view of the organization in the following words:

> If you are not seeking some miraculous, easy way to good mental health and are ready to make a business of it, and if you think you could help yourself if you only knew how to go about it, then welcome to Recovery, Inc.—it offers a systematic way to help yourself.[9]

There are no fees, although a free-will offering is taken at each meeting. One can make contact with a local chapter by consulting the telephone directory under Recovery, Inc. The national headquarters is located at 116 S. Michigan Avenue, Chicago, IL 60603.

**Emotions Anonymous.** Emotions Anonymous is another adaptation of Alcoholics Anonymous and is designed for anyone with emotional problems as defined by the individual who suffers. It ranges from people with minor bad habits to those who have suffered severe neuroses and have been hospitalized. The basic ingredients for the weekly group meetings are the same as those for Alcoholics Anonymous — public confession and group support. Between meetings a member is expected to practice more positive self-references, to read assigned literature, and to call a group leader if he or she experiences difficulty applying the principles of Emotions Anonymous. Some of the governing principles are as follows:

1. We, as members of Emotions Anonymous, offer the program and our personal stories of recovery and insight gained. This is all we do in helping others.

2. We *never* attempt to psychoanalyze a person or diagnose him.

3. We *never* argue with anyone or any group over his or their beliefs. They are welcome to their beliefs as we are welcome to ours. If they wish to follow the Emotions Anonymous program, that is their choice; they may still retain their other beliefs.

4. We *never* discuss religion, politics, national and international issues, or any other belief systems or policies. Emotions Anonymous has no opinion on outside issues.

5. Emotions Anonymous is a spiritual program but not a religious program. That is, it is not based on *any* formal system of religion. Anyone and everyone is welcome at Emotions Anonymous. There is room in Emotions for atheists, agnostics, and people of any faiths or of no faiths.

6. We only suggest a belief in a power greater than ourselves — "*God* as we understand Him." "God" may be considered to be a higher power, human love, a force for good, evolution, the motions of atoms, gravity — anything that has meaning to us.

7. We are friendly and warm to all people and make them welcome.

8. We never criticize anyone for anything. We do not judge. We look for the good and try to help bring it out.

9. We tell people how the program worked for us. We do not speak dogma and try to force our beliefs on other people.

10. The only purpose of Emotions Anonymous is to help us stay well ourselves and to help others to get well and stay well. We lose ourselves in this endeavor.[10]

The group believes that a selfish life is not worth living, and that love as expressed through social interest is the key to mental and emotional health. There is a 24-hour telephone answering service for people who need assistance. There are no dues or fees, but voluntary contributions are accepted. Contact may be made through the local telephone directory under Emotions Anonymous. The address for the national headquarters is P.O. Box 4245, Saint Paul, MN 55104. Telephone: (612) 647-9712.

## Parent Education Groups

Groups which are run by professionals for the purpose of teaching specialized coping skills and strategies are often called psychoeducational groups. Most of the parent education groups fall into this category. Some of the more helpful are discussed in the following pages.

**Parent Effectiveness Training Groups (PET).** This group is a profit-making program sponsored by Effectiveness Training Associates of Solana Beach, California. It is the brainchild of Thomas Gordon, Ph.D. and is based on humanistic psychology. Parent Effectiveness Training is the largest parenting group, having trained 8,000 instructors and 250,000 parents to date.

The program teaches parents to abandon power as a means of influencing the behavior of children. Children are to be treated with the respect normally accorded adults. Children do not misbehave; they merely behave in ways that are unacceptable to parents. Correct parenting is a matter of relating to children in such a way that the needs of both children and parents are respected. Three techniques are suggested for achieving this. When the child has a problem that does not conflict with the needs of the parent, *active listening* is recommended. Active listening is listening with deep understanding and responding in a way that lets the child know he is understood. No attempt is made to straighten the child out or to solve his or her problem. If the child's behavior interferes with a parent's needs, then *I-Messages* are used. Sending an I-Message is a matter of letting the child know how his behavior inconveniences the parent—"I am unable to concentrate on my reading as long as you continue to bounce that ball in here." It is assumed that the child will care enough about the parent to make the necessary adjustment in his behavior. If the child persists after an I-

Message, then a form of negotiation called the *no-lose method of problem-solving* becomes the appropriate technique. The program takes a respectful, optimistic view of human nature and the capacity to negotiate.

The course extends over eight to ten sessions; makes use of standard books, tapes, and charts; and costs between $50 and $90. You can make contact with a group leader through the local telephone directory under the listing Parent Effectiveness Training.

**Parent-Involvement Program.** Less well known is a program adapted from William Glasser's book *Reality Therapy.*[11] The key to the approach is involvement, which means establishing and maintaining a warm, honest, and affectionate relationship with children. Irresponsible behavior results from lack of respect for oneself, from seeing oneself as a failure. The antidote is to convince misbehaving children that they are prized, that someone cares about them—but without engaging in indulgence.

The seven steps in this program may be briefly summarized as follows:

1. Establish a warm, honest, affectionate relationship with the child largely through conversation on topics of mutual interest.

2. Help the child recognize what he is doing and accept responsibility for it.

3. Help the child judge the usefulness of such behavior in meeting his needs.

4. Help him set moderate, realistic goals for changing his behavior.

5. Press him gently for a commitment to his plan.

6. Accept no excuses—but allow for revisions of the plan based upon a reassessment of step 3.

7. Do not use the usual types of punishment but rather, use reasonable consequences that are agreed to by the child.

Glasser's Parent Involvement Program is less widely available to the public than is Gordon's Parent Effectiveness Training. Write William Glasser, M.D., at the Institute for Reality Therapy and Educator Training Center, Los Angeles, California, or contact the departments of psychology or counseling at the nearest university for information about the program.

**Adlerian Parenting Groups.** These groups, based upon Rudolph Dreikurs' book *Children: The Challenge,* differ from the two aforementioned groups in several respects.[12] It is assumed that misbehavior is really a misguided attempt to find one's place in the family, to gain a sense of belonging. The misbehaving child has usually been discouraged in his effort to find his place. All misbehavior is aimed at realizing one of four goals: (1) attention, (2) power, (3) revenge, or (4) overcoming inadequacy. The parent is taught to identify which of these goals the child is pursuing by analyzing his or her own emotional reaction to the child's misbehavior. Thereafter, the child is discouraged from dysfunctional behavior and encouraged to pursue a more enlightened approach. Emphasis is on cooperation and respect for the rights of others. There is also a heavy emphasis on independence training for children. It is important that they develop confidence in their own resources. The process of doing this is called encouragement.

It may be difficult to make contact with these groups, because they are not usually listed in the telephone directory. If you experience difficulty, write the Alfred Adler Institute, 333 Central Park West, New York, NY 10025.

**Active Parenting**. Active Parenting is a psychoeducational group based on the premise that effective parenting is learned parenting. Parents do not have to chart their own courses to successfully rear their children and provide a positive family environment. Rather, in Active Parenting they are encouraged to learn from the collected knowledge of the universe of other parents.

Active Parenting principles are presented to groups of approximately ten parents through videotapes that present structured lessons from the Active Parenting scheme. This approach fosters the creativity and initiative of the group, while the value of the group is enhanced by the quality education of each engaging presentation. Trained leaders and complementary literature offer additional group direction and resources.

Active parenting training is designed to turn defeated, confused parents into active, vigorous parents with confidence in themselves to resolve problems. Children, likewise, gain as their parents learn to understand, develop, and encourage them. The goal of Active Parenting is to create a cooperative, democratic family system where the growth of each member is prized. For more information on Active Parenting, write Active Parenting, 810 Franklin Court, SE, Marietta, GA 30067.

**Specialized Parent Groups**. Two parenting groups with more specialized purposes are Parents Without Partners and Parents Anonymous. Parents Without Partners is a national self-help group for single parents. It holds semimonthly meetings and has a calendar of family events for each day of the month. It publishes *Single Parent Magazine*, which is included in the $16 annual membership fee. The group is listed in the local telephone directory.

Parents Anonymous is designed to assist child abusers. It is similar in many respects to Alcoholics Anonymous in that it provides education and support. Weekly meetings are held and often free transportation and babysitting are provided. There is 24-hour telephone support. If a number is not listed in the local telephone directory, contact the national offices at 6738 South Sepulzeda Boulevard, Los Angeles, CA 90045, or call them at 1–800–421–0353.

**Additional Support Groups.** A perusal of a major newspaper yielded the following sample of the self-help groups which meet regularly in that city:

Adult Children of Dysfunctional Families
Adults with Learning Disabilities
Aging (groups for those who take care of the elderly)
Al-Anon, Alateen Family Groups
Alcoholics Anonymous
Alcohol and Drug Addiction
Alzheimer's Disease and Related Disorders Association
Couples Together
Gay Center "Coming Out"
Head Injury Recovery Center
Parents and Friends of Lesbians and Gays
Secular Organization for Sobriety (group for alcoholics who pre-
    fer a nonreligious approach)
Autism Society of America
Battered Women
Better Breathing Club
Bosom Buddies (an American Cancer Society group for breast
    cancer patients)
Cancer (groups for patients, family and friends)
Childless, Not By Choice (group for couples experiencing infer-
    tility or seeking to adopt children)
Chronic Pain Sufferers
Cocaine Anonymous
Co-Anon (for families and friends of cocaine users)
Co-Dependents Anonymous
Concern For Aging (for adult children with aging parents)
Compassionate Parents (for parents who have lost an infant)
Crime Victims
Depressive and Manic Depressive Association
Diabetes (for people with diabetes and their families)
Divorce Recovery
Divorce Support

Eating Disorders
Emotions Anonymous
Endometriosis
Epilepsy
Families and Friends of Homicide Victims
Families Caring for Older Adults
Fathers Are Parents Too (for single fathers)
Gamblers Anonymous
Gay Adult Children of Alcoholics
Georgia Alliance For the Mentally Ill
Georgia Association of Medical Victims (group for malpractice
    victims)
Grief Care (group for those who have experienced the death of a
    loved one)
Handicapped Organization for Women
Heart Menders (group for persons who have had heart attacks,
    strokes, or open heart surgery and their families)
Heart Transplants (pre- and post-transplant group meetings)
Incest Survivors
Learning Disabilities (group for parents and children with learn-
    ing disabilities)
Mothers of Persons With Aids
Mothers Without Custody
Multiple Sclerosis
Myasthenia Gravis Foundation
Ostomy Association
Overeaters Anonymous
Parents Anonymous
Phobia/Panic
PMS
S.A.D.S. (Seasonal Adjustment Disorder Syndrome) (group for
    persons who become depressed at seasonal time changes)

# The Genius of Self-help Groups

Although self-help groups differ greatly in their approaches, most seem to work well for many kinds of people. The key to the success of these groups may not lie in the particular program offered but, rather, in the motivation of persons who seek help from them. People who are willing to attend meetings, share testimonials of their successes and failures, and assist others to change are likely to be highly motivated to change themselves. If this is the case, then membership in these self-help groups may merely be a sign of the will to change rather than its cause. The authors, however, believe that the groups themselves provide a powerful stimulant for personal change—namely, the social reinforcement offered by group members who are committed to the same behavioral goals.

By definition, self-help groups motivate growth by combining the need to belong with the need for personal change. Katz and Bender state that self-help groups are "usually formed by peers who come together for mutual assistance in satisfying a common need, overcoming a common handicap or life-disrupting problem and bringing about social and/or personal change . . . . Self-help groups emphasize face to face social interactions and the assumption of personal responsibility by members."[13] Typically, the leadership of self-help groups comes from people who are experiencing, or who have experienced, the stressful conditions that bring the group together. There is much support from knowing that we are not alone nor unique in having a problem. To see others also battling with scourges such as alcoholism, compulsive overeating, loneliness, or the sense of failure that often accompanies divorce somehow makes the pain feel less unbearable. Moreover, the smiles, applause, and congratulations of friends who know what the problem is like can sustain motivation for personal change as little else can. The warmth, interest, and approval of others serve as organic fuel for our psyches. This social nourishment is likely the genius of these self-improvement groups.

The success of self-help groups also is determined by the group's collective health as a problem-solving unit and by the degree of cohesion achieved. Other characteristics cited as important to the effectiveness of these groups include:

- The opportunity to get help by helping others
- The willingness of group members to take risks
- The demystification of the member's life experiences
- Group consensus regarding a member's validity as a worthy human being
- Strong leadership from a leader willing to share leadership with others
- A focus on goals and the resolution of discrepancies in individual and group goals
- Active participation by group members
- Demand by the group for self-responsibility on the part of members
- The experience of a substitute culture in which identity changes can occur

Exhibit 8-3. Some Differences Between Self-help Groups and Therapy

| Parameters | Therapy | Versus | Self-help |
|---|---|---|---|
| Size of group | Limited | | Unlimited |
| Time commitment | Defined | | Undefined |
| Cost factor | Profit/nonprofit | | Nonprofit |
| Membership | Closed or open | | Open |
| Issues | Heterogenous | | Homogenous |
| Focus | Counseling | | Guidance |
| Politics | Apolitical | | Prepolitical |
| Goals | Emerging/changing | | Fixed |
| Activities | Reconstruction | | Reinforcement |
| Topics | Multiple | | Single theme |
| Leadership | Professional | | Lay |

- Expansion of alternative perceptions through continuous intervention

When considering self-help groups as an assist in coping with stressful life events, heed the following suggestions: Identify the benefits you are seeking and get clear on your expectations from the group prior to making your selection. Be aware that self-help groups have their own personalities and that a particular group may not match your personality. Remind yourself that self-help groups may be appropriate at some times but not at other times. Consider all of your alternatives for help.

## The Therapy Group Distinction

Whereas self-help groups are typically educational, problem-solving groups with a programmed structure and a focus on guidance, therapy groups adopt a free-flowing structure and emphasize self-exploration and interpersonal feedback. The goal in self-help groups is shared by all members and centers around a specific issue, whereas therapy groups pursue more general goals such as better mental health and self-actualization. Specific goals emerge and change among the members as a therapy group evolves. In self-help groups, the leader is usually a fellow sufferer. Therapy groups, in contrast, are led by trained professionals operating from a theoretical base. The therapy group leader emphasizes empathy and expertise. Exhibit 8-3 further depicts some of the differences between self-help groups and therapy groups.[14] Support groups fall somewhere between therapy and self-help groups in terms of these characteristics.

## The Informal Alliance

While self-help groups are helpful for certain kinds of problems, they may not be appropriate for others. Moreover, a particular kind of self-help group may not exist in our community. In any event we may wish to strengthen our resolve for personal change by deliberately choosing to spend time with people who will serve as an inspiration for the desired change. In this way we use the well-established habits of others to develop similar ones.

Parents show awareness of the influence of others when they encourage their children to associate with superior students. Likewise there is much folklore that tells of the woeful story of people of good character turning bad out of attraction for people of ill-fame. Translated into practical terms, this means that, if you are trying to stop the drinking habit, do not ride home with a friend who normally stops at the local bar; rather, seek out the company of people not addicted to drinking. If you are having trouble getting to work on time, drive with friends who arrive in plenty of time. If you are trying to lose weight, eat lunch with the gang that takes the salad-and-yogurt route. If you are trying to exercise more, join a neighbor who jogs each evening. If you are trying to stop smoking, associate with others who have kicked the habit. Carefully selected company is a marvelous way of boosting the resolve to change.

Not only is company important when trying to make changes in behavior, it is at least equally important as a source of nurturance and support for daily living. We need the goodwill, warmth, and intimacy of others as much as we need food and sleep. Lack of human support soon shows in our energy level. Unfortunately, many people have wired themselves into relationships that sap their energy. Negative people are like bloodsuckers—they literally leave us tired and discouraged.

Spouses, parents, or friends sometimes serve as our therapists. The amount of sustenance that some gain from friends and family members is truly incredible. Unfortunately, we seldom recognize the importance of these relationships because they are so constant. Remove them, however, and we feel as though our legs have been cut off. If these relationships are so vital to our psychic well-being, then we should be prepared to invest richly in their maintenance and improvement.

There are some hazards, of course, in using friends and loved ones in this therapeutic manner. If we admit them to the inner circle of our psyches, we are somewhat vulnerable. Confidants may not carefully respect confidentiality, or they may use a disclosure to increase their own power base. These risks pall, however, when compared with the withering of the human spirit that results from lack of intimacy.

# Seeking Professional Assistance

In addition to using our own resources or those of lay self-help groups, at times we may be in need of assistance from a professional helper. Even in such cases, we are still exercising self-management, since it is up to each of us to choose the form of professional therapy. Unfortunately, most people stumble into their contacts with therapists. They seldom inquire in depth about the training or kind of treatment used by the professional. Usually they depend on a recommendation from a friend or casually choose a name from the Yellow Pages. This is merely a form of Russian roulette. The effects of therapy can range from helpful to hurtful. Since choosing a therapist is a serious matter, there are a few considerations that may make one's selection a more profitable one.

## Become Acquainted with Available Resources

Be aware of the differences among mental health workers, since they vary in occupational affiliation, work setting, degree of specialization, theoretical orientation, techniques, and personality. Psychiatrists differ from other mental health workers primarily in that they are licensed to practice medicine. This means that they can prescribe psychotropic medications such as tranquilizers, sedatives, and antidepressants. This can sometimes be an advantage, since chemical assistance can prove valuable for some people. Medication can impede therapy, however, if used as a substitute for the more permanent effects of self-examination and the building of a repertoire of coping skills. Skillful psychiatrists will use psychotropic medication as an adjunct to, rather than a substitute for, psychotherapy. Other mental health workers include clinical psychologists, counseling psychologists, psychiatric social workers, and counselors. Clinical and counseling psychologists usually hold a doctorate. Psychiatric social workers usually have a masters degree as do counselors.

There are significant differences in the work settings of mental health practitioners. The basic breakdown is between public and private services. The one clear difference between settings is the amount of money therapy will cost—seeking therapy at a public clinic, for example, is significantly less expensive than is private counseling. Sources of low-cost aid are community mental health centers, college counseling centers, family and child service centers, schools, and state rehabilitation agencies.

Professionals also differ in regard to specialization. While the majority conduct general practice, some therapists specialize in family therapy; others, in sex therapy; and yet others, in group therapy. Group therapy, which costs about half that of individual therapy, is often a sound choice because it offers the additional dimension of reality that is provided by other group members, frequently, the most helpful insight will come from them. In our opinion the social nature of group treatment makes it less provincial and more representative of the real world. Group leaders vary widely in their approaches, and as with other forms of therapy, the effect on a participant may be good, neutral, or bad.

Mental health practitioners also differ in regard to theoretical positions. These differences stem in part from variation in the types of clients seen by the various mental health workers, but they also indicate sharp differences in their views of the causes of human problems. Differences in theoretical orientations result in differences in technique. Although there is some reason to believe that the depth of a therapist's experience, rather than the therapist's theoretical background, is more likely to determine the technique, it is, nevertheless, quite likely that theory also influences practice.[15] Consequently, it is important to ascertain a therapist's theoretical orientation before beginning therapy. While there are many therapeutic approaches, most fall nicely into one of two broad categories: those seeking to alter personality and those seeking to alter behavior.

Most counseling theories are of the personality-altering varieties. These theories assume that basic, internal personality flaws cause specific behavioral symptoms. The goal of therapy is to attack these basic causes in order to restructure the personality. The basic cause may be an imbalance between warring aspects of the personality, an inadequate self-concept, an overly oppressive conscience, lack of meaning, or an inferiority complex. Moreover, these theories assume that behavioral symptoms will disappear once the basic cause of a disease is removed. In this type of theory, the self-exploration stage of counseling is likely to be extensive, as it is necessary to establish and change the dynamics responsible for the personality disturbance. Symptoms are not usually dealt with directly; the therapist assumes they would merely be replaced by others if the basic disease is not cured.

Therapists who seek to alter behavior are generally more limited in their goals. Unlike the personality-altering types, behavior-oriented therapists assume no basic disease and, consequently, take symptoms more seriously. They believe that symptoms are learned and that, therefore, they can be unlearned. They design a direct frontal attack upon the symptoms.

These therapists believe that the causes of problem behaviors are all in a person's present situation. They are less interested in experiences out of the distant past that might be construed to be responsible for present behavior. They are more interested in the present conditions in a person's life that trigger and maintain a behavior. These therapists engineer changes in a person's situation where possible. They may attempt to teach new social skills, rid the person of dysfunctional fears, or reinforce more appropriate behavior or thoughts. In this type of therapy, one is likely to be far busier outside the counseling session than one would be in personality-altering therapies. Since goals are more limited with this kind of therapy, fewer sessions are likely to be necessary.

The therapist's personality is likely to be a significant factor. In a well-controlled experiment with encounter groups, the ideal group leaders were identified as being moderate in stimulating others to participate and in controlling the group, high in caring and warmth, and high in assisting clients in understanding what was happening to them. This ability to help clients understand the meaning of their own experiences was more closely associated with productive outcomes than was any other single trait.[16]

The ability to understand the meaning of a client's experience involves accurate empathy. Most experts agree that accurate empathy, genuineness, and nonpossessive warmth form a trilogy of traits that characterize a good therapist.[17]

## Get the Specifics Before Beginning

We have a right to ask questions of a therapist before committing ourselves to treatment. This reduces the likelihood of future disillusionment. There is a clear relationship between success in therapy and the degree to which counselor and client hold common expectations for the therapeutic process.[18] The Public Citizen's Health Research Group, one of Ralph Nader's groups, suggests forty-one questions a potential client might put to a potential therapist.[19] While most of the questions are helpful in getting a good reading on the therapist, the total seems a bit too much. Persisting with such a lengthy questionnaire is likely to trigger the ire of professionals, and indeed, this is precisely what happened when the Health Research Group sent out 1,990 questionnaires to psychiatrists, psychologists, and psychiatric social workers in the Washington, D.C., area. Only 348 were returned. A few well-chosen questions, however, are likely to be answered courteously by most professionals, and the resulting information should prove helpful.

We might begin such an inquiry by stating: "If I commit myself to the process of therapy, I want to feel good about it, and it would help me to know a few things about you and the kind of experiences I am likely to be letting myself in for. Would you mind answering a few questions that are very important to me?" Such an approach is likely to receive a generous response from most professionals. Perhaps the most telling test would be for the professional to become defensive and to refuse to respond our questions. We may wish to raise questions about the following:

- The therapist's credentials, training, and years of experience.
- Theoretical orientation (be sure to ask what this means in terms of treatment).
- The kinds of things that are likely to happen in therapy.
- Financial arrangements, including (a) amount of time per session, (b) cost per session, (c) an estimate of the number of sessions that might be required, (d) when payment is due, and (e) penalties that might be assessed for a missed appointment.

Nader's group recommends drawing up a formal contract with all the above considerations and many more. Once again, this action may be more harmful than helpful to the therapeutic relationship, at least in the eyes of many professionals. Still, asking questions informally about the concerns mentioned is likely to put our minds at rest and, therefore, to facilitate a higher degree of trust in the relationship.

## Therapy by the Book

Bibliotherapy, also called bibliocounseling, refers to a type of therapy where the patient is assigned certain topics, books, or articles for the understanding or insight that they will bring to his or her therapeutic need. People most likely have used bibliotherapy as long as the printed word has been available. In fact, a sign over the library door in ancient Thebes, Greece proclaimed it "The Healing Place of the Soul."

Reading has a tremendous influence upon people. The results vary, however, from person to person. What may be inspiring and soothing to one person may evoke anxiety and defensiveness in another. For example, most of us have experienced the medical student syndrome, wherein we mysteriously notice the symptoms of a disease in ourselves after having read about it.

While there are no prescriptive guides that can unerringly direct a reader to sources of books guaranteed to bring about intended effects, careful selection can be important. For example, one leading executive-development firm routinely assigns *The Godfather* to clients whom they feel have difficulty facing the hard realities of the business world.[20] They assign *Business as a Game* to clients lacking an appreciation for the way in which one succeeds in the business world.[21] Some therapists prescribe books by philosophers. The philotherapeutic approach is based on the assumption that most troubles encountered today have been addressed in the treatises of philosophers throughout the ages. Increasingly, therapists of all persuasions are supplementing the effects of their weekly sessions by homework assignments that quite often include prescribed reading.

For example, a 1987 survey by one of the authors of 138 mental health service practitioners in one large metropolitan area, indicated that 87 percent were using bibliotherapy. These professionals were asked to list the titles of the books they most frequently assigned to their clients. The number of books totaled 377, with 99 being mentioned by more than one professional. These practitioners stated that the books were assigned for both their content and their therapeutic value. For example, the practitioners commented that bibliotherapy was useful in helping clients process ideas that were foreign to them, in helping clients work on issues between sessions, and in assisting the therapist in understanding the client's issues when the reading assignment was met with resistance. There was an awareness that reading assignments were not well suited for everyone, and it was the therapist's job to insure a good match. Books listed most frequently by the respondents appear in Exhibit 8–4. Exhibit 8–5 contains a longer list of the books cited by at least three respondents.

The authors wish to share several sources that have proven helpful to their clients. While there are literally hundreds of appropriate volumes, the following ones have been chosen for their wide range of appeal. The reader can easily find many other useful books in each of the following categories. The books in this chapter have been selected for (1) their readability and general interest values, (2) their widespread use by therapists, (3) references to them in the professional literature, (4) their timeless quality, and (5) their availability.

## Negotiation in Marriage

Maladjustment in marriage often centers around patterns associated with the meeting of power and sexual needs. In every arena participants want to be involved in the decision-making process; marriages are no exception.

John Narcisco and David Burkett's book *Declare Yourself: Discovering the Me in Relationships* analyzes the basis for negotiation in interpersonal relationships.[22] In many marriages one person plays the role of the Demander, while the other acts the part of the Deferrer. Even in marriages with an egalitarian base, one partner often makes more demands than the other. Most of the time the slight imbalance creates no discernible strain on the marriage; however, if demands become excessive, Deferrers in time begin to resent their position. If the resentment becomes severe enough, the Deferrer may defect, that is, begin unconsciously to make extensive use of suffering, depression, or anger to strengthen his or her power base in the marriage. Suffering, depression, and anger can be attention-getting behaviors. The book suggests negotiation alternatives designed to lessen the Demander-Deferrer struggle in marital interaction.

**Exhibit 8-4.** Books Most Frequently Used by Therapists

| Book | Times Listed |
|---|---|
| *Women Who Love Too Much* | 31 |
| *Adult Children of Alcoholics* | 19 |
| *The Road Less Traveled* | 19 |
| *What Color is Your Parachute?* | 19 |
| *I'm O.K., You're O.K.* | 13 |
| *Passages* | 13 |
| *Peoplemaking* | 13 |
| *I'll Quit Tomorrow* | 9 |
| *It Will Never Happen To Me* | 9 |
| *The Struggle for Intimacy* | 9 |
| *When I Say No I Feel Guilty* | 9 |
| *The Art of Loving* | 8 |

*(Text continued on page 241)*

**Exhibit 8-5.** Books Counselors Use in Bibliotherapy Listed by Topic

---

**Adult Children of Alcoholics**

Beattie, M. 1987. *Codependent No More: How to Stop Controlling Others and Start Caring for Yourself.* New York: Harper & Row.

Black, C. 1987. *It Will Never Happen to Me.* New York: Ballantine Books.

Woititz, J. G. 1983. *Adult Children of Alcoholics.* Pompano Beach, Florida: Health Communications.

**Abuse / Sexual & Physical**

Brady, K. 1981. *Father's Days: A True Story of Incest.* New York: Dell Publishing.

McNaron, T. A., and Morgan, Y., eds. 1982. *Voices in the Night.* Pittsburgh: Cleis Press.

**Adolescent Issues**

Loughmiller, C. 1965. *Wilderness Road.* Austin, Texas: Hogg Foundation of Mental Health, University of Texas.

**Anger**

Rubin, T. 1987. *The Angry Book.* New York: Collier.

**Assertiveness**

Alberti, R. E., and Emmons, M. L. 1978. *Your Perfect Right: A Guide to Assertive Behavior* (3rd ed.). San Luis Obispo, California: Impact.

Bloom, L., Coburn, K., and Pearlman, J. 1976. *The New Assertive Woman.* New York: Dell Publishing.

**Career**

Bolles, R. 1988. *What Color is Your Parachute?.* Berkeley, California: Ten Speed Press.

**Chemical Dependency**

Alcoholics Anonymous. 1953. *Twelve Steps and Twelve Traditions.* New York: Alcoholics Anonymous World Services, Inc.

Larson, E. 1985. *Stage Two Recovery: Life Beyond Addiction.* New York: Harper & Row.

Milam, J. R., and Ketcham, K. 1981. *Under the Influence: A Guide to the Myths and Realities of Alcoholism.* Seattle: Madrona.

Woititz, J. G. 1985. *The Struggle for Intimacy.* Pompano Beach, Florida: Health Communications.

**Children of Alcoholics**

Black, C. 1982. *My Dad Loves Me, My Dad Has a Disease.* Denver: MAC Printing and Publications.

---

*(Continued on next page)*

**Exhibit 8-5.** (Continued)

---

## Cognitive Therapy
Ellis, A., and Harper, R. A. 1975. *A New Guide to Rational Living.* Englewood Cliffs, New Jersey: Prentice-Hall.
Glasser, W. 1975. *Reality Therapy.* New York: Harper & Row.

## Communication
Howe, R. L. 1963. *The Miracle of Dialogue.* New York: Harper & Row.
Satir, V. 1972. *Peoplemaking.* Palo Alto, California: Science and Behavior Books.

## Death
Kubler-Ross, E. 1970. *On Death and Dying.* New York: Macmillan.

## Depression
Burns, D. 1980. *Feeling Good: The New Mood Therapy.* New York: Morrow.
Frankl, V. 1984. *Man's Search for Meaning.* New York: Touchstone Books.

## Developmental
Crabb, L. 1988. *Inside Out.* Colorado Springs: NavPress.
Peck, M. S. 1985. *The Road Less Traveled.* New York: Simon & Schuster.
Sheahy, G. 1977. *Passages.* New York: Bantam Books.

## Divorce
Gardner, R. 1971. *The Boys and Girls Book About Divorce.* New York: Bantam Books.
Trafford, A. 1984. *Crazy Time: Surviving Divorce.* New York: Bantam Books.

## Eating Disorders
Hollis, J. 1986. *Fat Is a Family Affair.* New York: Harper & Row.
Orbach, S. 1987. *Fat Is a Feminist Issue.* New York: Berkley Publishing Group.

## Family Issues
Bradshaw J. 1988. *Bradshaw on: The Family.* Deerfield Beach, Florida: Health Communications.
Napier, A., and Whitaker, C. 1980. *The Family Crucible.* New York: Bantam Books.
Satir, V. 1982. *Conjoint Family Therapy* (3rd ed.). Palo Alto, California: Science and Behavior Books.

## Grief
Viorst, J. 1987. *Necessary Losses.* New York: Fawcett Book Group.

---

*(Continued on next page)*

**Exhibit 8-5.** (Continued)

---

**Male Issues**
Kiley, D. 1984. *The Peter Pan Syndrome*. New York: Avon Books.
Zilbergeld, B. 1978. *Male Sexuality*. New York: Bantam Books.


**Marriage**
Bach, G., and Wyden, P. 1981. *The Intimate Enemy*. New York: Avon Books.
Crabb, L. 1982. *Marriage Builder: A Blueprint for Couples and Counselors.*
  Grand Rapids: Zondervan.
Schwartz, R., and Schwartz, L. 1986. *Becoming a Couple*. Lanham, Maryland:
  University Press of America.


**Motivation**
Dyer, W. 1980. *The Sky's the Limit*. New York: Simon & Schuster.


**Parenting**
Dreikurs, R., and Soltz, V. 1964. *Children: The Challenge*. New York:
  Hawthorn/Dutton.
Gordon, T. 1970. *Parent Effectiveness Training*. New York: P. H. Wyden.


**Relationships**
Harris, T. 1982. *I'm OK, You're OK*. New York: Avon Books.
Napier, A. 1988. *Fragile Bond: In Search of an Equal, Intimate & Enduring
  Bond*. New York: Harper & Row.
Powell, J. 1974. *Secret of Staying in Love*. Valencia, CA: Tabor Publishing.
Powell, J. 1969. *Why Am I Afraid to Tell You Who I Am*. Valencia, CA: Tabor
  Publishing.
Smith, M. 1985. *When I Say No I Feel Guilty*. New York: Bantam Books.


**Sex**
Carnes, P. 1983. *Sexual Addiction*. Minneapolis: CompCare Publications.
Wheat, E., and Wheat, G. 1981. *Intended for Pleasure*. Old Tappan, New
  Jersey: F. H. Revell.


**Spiritual**
Seamands, D. A. 1981. *Healing for Damaged Emotions*. Wheaton, Illinois:
  Victor Books.


**Women's Issues**
Gilligan, C. 1982. *In a Different Voice*. Cambridge, Massachusetts: Harvard
  University Press.
Norwood, R. 1985. *Women Who Love Too Much*. Los Angeles, California: J.
  P. Tarcher.

---

*(Text continued from page 237)*

George Bach and Peter Wyden's *The Intimate Enemy: How to Fight Fair in Love and Marriage* views the universal traits of aggression and hostility between marital partners as healthy, growth-producing phenomena.[23] Their premise is that all human beings have aggressive and hostile feelings and that to expect these to be shelved in marital interactions is not only unrealistic but damaging to understanding and growth in the relationship. Indeed, genuine intimacy can only be achieved through therapeutic aggression, and the authors present a set of guidelines for engaging in "constructive fighting."

Another book frequently assigned by marriage counselors is *The Mirages of Marriage* by William Lederer and Don Jackson.[24] The authors take the position, based on experience and statistical evidence, that within a few months of the wedding most marriages are a severe disappointment to the partners. They blame faulty assumptions for the ensuing unhappiness and, in a highly readable fashion, present an appealing and conclusive explanation of a systems approach to marriage. Marriage is seen as more than the sum of the personalities of the participants and, therefore, troubles that occur cannot be explained by examining each spouse. Rather, it is the system generated as the result of the interaction of these two personalities that needs to be understood and confronted.

The authors examine seven false assumptions that people consciously or unconsciously bring with them to the altar. For example, "Love is necessary for a satisfactory marriage" is an assumption challenged on the basis that spouses often confuse romance with love and are torn apart when the essentially selfish promises of romance are not fulfilled.

Most of the literature on marriage seems to imply that, once married, a couple must work it out, although statistics dramatically refute such a prescription. Simply put, many marriages are just not meant to be. Moreover, the legal and emotional commitment of marriage often leaves divorced people exhausted, confused, and guilt-ridden at having failed in a major life endeavor. Mel Krantzler's *Creative Divorce* turns such an attitude around and examines the positive and creative opportunities afforded by divorce.[25] Everybody knows that there is a fine line in judging whether a marriage is "good" or "bad" or whether a couple should stay together or divorce. No simple formula is available to make that line vividly discernible, but Krantzler's book clearly helps those individuals who have resolved in their own minds that their marriage is no longer tenable. It also helps the reader to handle loneliness and the effects of divorce on children.

## Sexual Adjustment

Although the bumper sticker that proclaims "Give me the old days, when the air was clean and sex was dirty" describes some people's reactions to the current sexual revolution, few refute the notion that correct information regarding sexual functions is important. Fred Belliveau and Lin Richter's *Understanding Human Sexual Inadequacy* outlines much of the voluminous research done by Masters and Johnson.[26] The reader who is interested in an informative and fairly thorough summary of the causes of sexual failure will find much information in this volume. It is well written and tries to capture the psychological and social components of sexual functioning as they relate to the physical side.

*The New Our Bodies, Ourselves: The Book by and for Women* is the sequel to an unusual and appealing grass-roots version of women's liberation at its best.[27] It began when a group of Boston women, frustrated by their experiences with physicians, talked and shared information with each other. The collective realization of how little they knew about their bodies led them to believe that such ignorance was probably widespread. The result was an earlier book, which this version updates. The new version has a comprehensive treatment of the physiological aspects of sexual and reproductive functions and also several sections on general health and nutrition.

The volume encourages openness and stresses the importance of getting and giving psychological support. In that spirit it necessarily includes a wide representation of value systems. Some readers may take exception to some parts, which seem to flaunt conventional mores; nonetheless, the volume is a storehouse of information not readily available elsewhere.

The sexual awakening of adolescents leaves many adults puzzled regarding their roles. Adults' recollections of adolescence are frequently meaningless, confusing, or painful, and the current trends in sexual values compete heavily for an adolescent's attention. Sol Gordon's *The Sexual Adolescent: Communication with Teenagers About Sex* is expressly written to help parents and professionals become knowledgeable regarding current sexual issues and to be effective in discussing these with teenagers.[28] Sol Gordon squarely sides with the camp that believes teenagers are going to make their own sexual decisions, and that the responsibility of adults is to be available, knowledgeable, and communicative. He pleads for parental openness and honesty regarding sexual matters, and he intensively strives to make the reader aware of the questions teenagers have on their minds, whether or not they are asking them. The finer points of sexual morality are not avoided, but the emphasis is clearly on the more pragmatic issues of venereal diseases, unwanted children, and exploitative sex. Included is a glossary of sexual slang and a bibliography.

Another excellent book, by the veteran psychologist-sex educator James McCary, is *A Complete Sex Education for Parents, Teenagers, and Young Adults*.[29] All of McCary's writings on sex are dispassionate and scholarly but are extremely engaging and readable. This volume is outstanding in that it offers parents an accurate accounting of social and sexual issues with a minimum of moral judgment. As such, it can be used as a catalyst for family discussion. The recounting of the mechanics of sex is complete and nontechnical. The varieties of sexual behaviors are examined, and common myths and fallacies are rebutted by facts. This book is also a fine resource for any young couple contemplating marriage.

## Parenting

Parents are frequently hounded and tormented by their own consciences for presumed faults regarding child-rearing. However hard they try, there always seems to be something else they could or should do, or should have done, in behalf of their offspring. Worse still, there never seem to be clear answers to the really critical issues: how much guidance to offer children, how much to require of them—and in what areas of their lives—how much to involve them in participatory management of family decisions, how open to be regarding sensitive topics, and the like.

Gerald Patterson applied behavioral theory to child management in the programmed text, *Living with Children*.[30] It is based on the acknowledgment that people learn most of their behavior from other people. The book shows parents how to encourage desirable behavior and gradually eliminate undesirable behavior in their children. It offers step-by-step advice on handling such things as, "The Child Who Fights Too Often," "The 'I Don't Want To' Child," "The Overly Active, Noisy Child," " The Frightened Child," and "The Withdrawn Child." The principles are simple, easily understood, and likely to work *if they are used*. This handle on these child-management problems has given security and direction to many befuddled parents.

## Vocational Adjustment

Our life work is perhaps the most important issue to be resolved, with the possible exception of matters relating to marriage and family. How do we best integrate interests, abilities, and opportunities? How do we know what rewards to expect of a vocation before we commit ourselves to long years of preparation? These and many other similar questions constitute legitimate concerns for both youth and adults.

Libraries are filled with books about working, yet the hapless reader searching the stacks for vocational insights will be disappointed more often than not. *What Color Is Your Parachute? A Practical Manual for Job-Hunters and Career Changers* by Richard Nelson Bolles delivers its readers from such anguish.[31] Bolles has organized the methods and materials of vocational guidance into a highly readable and especially useful resource. He starts from the premise that getting a job can be a lot of work and then organizes the tasks and resources available to the career planner. How to find jobs, practical hints on getting a job, building a second career, a directory called "Help," which lists many free or inexpensive aids, and information on counseling agencies are just some of the topics included in the book. The bibliography is particularly helpful. Using it, a serious career planner can divide the task into subgoals and find books about interviewing, skill analysis, or even what to do when fired. Working and career planning are complex matters, and this volume successfully undercuts the part that chance plays and touts deliberate and intelligent job choices. This book is revised annually so the reader should be careful to get the most up-to-date volume.

Another volume that can be helpful is John Holland's *Making Vocational Choices: A Theory of Careers.*[32] Holland posits the existence of six personality types—realistic, investigative, artistic, social, enterprising, and conventional—that provide the bases for determining which environments and types of people are most likely to be suited to each other. Holland believes that most people can provide their own vocational guidance if they are exposed to the proper resources. Included in the book is the "Self-Directed Search," a self-administering, self-scoring, and self-interpreting questionnaire. Upon completion of the questionnaire, one arrives at a three-letter code that represents a blend of the personality types. Using this code, an individual then turns to the Occupations Finder, a classification section that lists the occupational areas that are likely to be rewarding to the personality type. Readers are encouraged to begin their occupational investigations with the job areas that fit their individual personalities.

## Handling Stress

Many people are so exhausted by chronic anxiety and other forms of sress that they have little energy left to devote to the pleasurable pursuits of life. Consequently, they feel that life is passing them by, that they are so squeezed by the worries of the future and the regrets of the past that they do not have a present. It is difficult to concentrate, to attend, to be truly present with others. The ability to relax, as well as to cope effectively with mental feverishness, is a serious problem.

Hans Selye, perhaps the greatest living expert on stress, has written two volumes on the subject. His epic work, *The Stress of Life,* greatly influenced the medical world's understanding of psychosomatic illnesses.[33] Another volume, *Stress Without Distress*, offers a prescription for minimizing psychic insults to the nervous system and suggests ways of using stress to achieve a rewarding lifestyle.[34] In both volumes Selye convincingly demonstrates the physiological effects of coping with high stress. He explains these effects as stemming from the General Adaptation Syndrome. He suggests that we have a limited amount of adaptive energy for coping, and when it is exhausted, death is a certainty. The rest of the volume is concerned with creative adjustments that conserve this precious energy. Reading these volumes is apt to cause the reader to recognize the futility and utter wastefulness of many habits.

Harvard professor Herbert Benson, M.D., has written a best-seller entitled *The Relaxation Response*.[35] Benson is one of the world's leading researchers on relaxation. Part of his research was conducted in his laboratory and part was conducted in the library, reading the vast amount of literature on meditation. He became convinced that meditative practices in Hinduism, Buddhism, Sufism, Taoism, Judaism, and Christianity all triggered identical physiological and psychological conditions. Each of these meditative practices activated the Relaxation Response, a protective mechanism that turns off harmful bodily effects created by overstress. It decreases heart rate, lowers metabolism, decreases rate of breathing, and restores a healthier balance to the body. The practice combines patterned breathing, muscle relaxation, and meditation in a simple, effortless exercise that requires 15 to 20 minutes, once or twice daily. Benson concludes that the physiologic changes elicited by this technique are similar to those induced by Transcendental Mediation, Zen, yoga, autogenic training, progressive relaxation, and hypnosis. Millions of people have found that some form of these techniques significantly helps in reducing nervousness and stress. In a later volume, *Beyond the Relaxation Response*, Benson stresses the importance of the "faith factor" for achieving contentment and relaxation.[36]

## Asserting Oneself

Many people live with self-contempt because they feel unable to stand up for their rights. It seems that others make all their decisions. They feel overwhelmed by the forcefulness of others. Worse still, they feel frightened and even guilty when they try to assert themselves. They are unsure of their rights. They confuse self-respect with selfishness. Being unskillful and uncertain of their rights, they equivocate in expressing their preferences, and others find it quite easy to overrule them.

Robert Alberti and Michael Emmons have written a highly readable book on assertiveness, entitled *Your Perfect Right: A Guide to Assertive Living*.[37] Early chapters assist the reader in overcoming guilt feelings about legitimate forms of self-assertion. Later chapters contain vignettes showing when assertive behavior is appropriate and offer examples of nonassertive, aggressive, and assertive responses to these situations. The book is useful in realigning thinking about our right to assert ourselves and in providing illustrative examples of good taste in assertiveness.

More comprehensive than the Alberti and Emmons book, *I Am Worth It* by Jan Kelley and Barbara Winship contains a three-part assertive response. It consists of empathy, conflict, and action.[38] Very simply, it means that we should let others know that their views are understood and also share with them our own thinking about a matter. Finally we should tell others what is going to happen (if it is our choice) or what we would like to see happen (if it is another's choice). The use of this complete response pattern is respectful of the feelings of others and likely to make the assertive response effective and nonhurtful to the relationship.

Arnold Lazarus and Allen Fay, in *I Can If I Want To,* attack twenty nonfunctional beliefs common to American culture that effectively inhibit people from asserting themselves.[39] Beliefs such as "I am a victim of circumstances," "I must earn happiness," and "I must please other people to get along in this world" contribute to a feeling of powerlessness and worthlessness. These feelings, in turn, discourage us from sending clear signals to others about opinions, preferences, and values. Consequently, we are inadequate in negotiating with others for our wants and needs because we fail to communicate directly to others what we really want.

The authors identify basic erroneous themes that tend to ruin lives, reveal the faulty assumptions behind these themes, suggest a basis for more functional thinking about them, and prescribe corrective behavior. As an example, they suggest that we counter the belief that we are a helpless victim of circumstances by asking these questions: If I were offered $10,000 in cash to do the thing I say I can't do, would I do it? If a child of mine or the person closest to me were kidnapped and I knew that I would never see this person alive again if I didn't do the thing I say I can't do, would I do it? Answering such questions leads us to change "I can't" statements to "I choose to" statements and helps us to recognize that we can do what we will, that we can do most things we want to do if willing to pay the price. This work is an ingenious and spirited book that has proved helpful to many people as they identified the common themes that have created tension and unhappiness in their lives.

In his book, *When I Say No, I Feel Guilty,* Manuel J. Smith presents several techniques to enable people to respond assertively to criticism and manipulative statements.[40] One technique, Broken Record, involves repeating a request or wish for as long as necessary in a calm, relaxed voice while ignoring all side issues brought up by a critic. Fogging involves accepting manipulative criticism by calmly acknowledging the probability that there may be some truth in the criticism while clearly maintaining the right to do what we want to about behavior. Negative Assertion is a matter of accepting responsibility for mistakes without apologizing for them. In Negative Inquiry, we invite further critical statements repeatedly until the other person is required to see the real basis for the criticism. And Self-Disclosure involves initiating and accepting discussion of both the positive and negative aspects of our personality in order to encourage honest communication and to reduce manipulation and defensiveness. The brief descriptions of these techniques do not do them justice; Smith's forceful writing style and powerful illustrations make his techniques come alive on the printed page. The book is highly recommended for people besieged with constant criticism from salespeople, casual acquaintances, business contacts, and others who are relatively unimportant to them.

Andrew Salter was one of the first to draw attention to the lack of assertiveness on the part of neurotics. In his book, *Conditioned Reflex Therapy*, he faults conditioning by parents and society in general for nonassertive lifestyles.[41] In the desire to be accepted and liked by everyone, people become self-conscious, apologetic, and afraid of inconveniencing people. What appears to be courtesy becomes a fraud—we defer only because we are afraid of making others angry.

Salter suggests six ways to become a more assertive person: (1) become emotionally outspoken, expressing likes and dislikes, annoyance, regret, love, and other emotions; (2) show emotions by facial expressions; (3) contradict and attack when in disagreement rather than simulate agreeability; (4) use the word "I" as much as possible; (5) express agreement when praised; and (6) begin to act more spontaneously. While some of these suggestions may appear to be overcompensations in the opposite direction, Salter presumes that the reader's current tendency toward an inhibited lifestyle will result in a healthy compromise.

## Lack of Meaning

Many people are plagued from time to time with a feeling that their lives lack meaning. While some people appear to spend little time trying to resolve these questions, others are made restless by the need to relate themselves to their social and physical worlds, They tirelessly seek to construct a personal cosmology.

Victor Frankl's book *Man's Search For Meaning* has been used by many therapists whose clients are unable to find personal meaning in life.[42] Frankl, who suffered the travails of Auschwitz, impresses the reader in an unassuming way with his ideas regarding the meaning of life and the suffering people endure in the pursuit of meaningful lives. Most people are repelled by the thought or act of suicide, but Frankl asks, "*Why* don't you commit suicide?" Each individual has his own unique answer to this question, and in this answer are found the beginnings of meaning and purpose in life.

The search for meaning in life leads people to create systems of belief. In *The Religions of Man* Huston Smith has written one of the clearer and fairer accounts of the world's great religions: Hinduism, Buddhism, Confucianism, Taoism, Islam, Judaism, and Christianity.[43] Explained simply and sympathetically are the reasons that each of these religions has attracted millions of devout followers. While we are not interested in sponsoring any one religious position, we do realize that some readers may be in search of a more satisfying world view that can add meaning to their everyday lives, and a review of major religions may prove helpful.

# Depression

For many people, depression is as uncontrollable as an eclipse of the sun. One's energy dips along with one's mood. Interest in appearance, sex, work, and community sags markedly. Feelings of guilt, worthlessness, and hopelessness mysteriously wash in like waves. Relations with others suffer enormously, and the joy of living evaporates. For some, the greatest battle of their lives is with this dreaded ogre called depression.

*The New Guide to Rational Living* by Albert Ellis and Robert Harper challenges habits of self-criticism.[44] Most people are their own worst enemies because they demand things of themselves and others that are unreasonable and often just plain stupid. The natural outcome of continual self-criticism is depression, and the cause of such a habit can be found in the faulty, negative self-talk people engage in so frequently. Ellis attacks the assumptions upon which most depressing self-statements are based. He tries to convince readers that, for example, it is ridiculous indeed to believe that we must be loved by everyone. But, if so, why do we often act as if life is dreadful when someone expresses dislike? Such conclusions are reached by most people because of a faulty mechanism in their systems of logical reasoning that betrays them time and again in their daily lives. Ellis helps the reader to redefine a system of logic so that helpful and satisfying conclusions about daily events and interpersonal relationships can lead to more functional and positive feelings.

## Self-worth

Related to depression is concern about personal worth. Many people run their lives as if they were on a neurotic treadmill, running like crazy to try to prove their self-worth. Inferiority feelings are extremely common. Although all people experience the haunting pain of such feelings from time to time, some people's lives are governed by an attempt to gain parity or superiority.

Thomas Harris, in *I'm OK—You're OK*, applies the principles of transactional analysis to the development of self-worth.[45] He analyzes four life positions underlying behavior: the immature person's anxious dependence, expressed as "I'm not OK—You're OK"; the despairing position, called "I'm not OK—You're not OK"; the criminal position, called "I'm OK—You're not OK"; and the mature position, expressed as "I'm OK—You're OK."

He helps the reader examine the effect of his communication on others by drawing attention to three active facets in our personalities: the Parent personifies the "do's" and "don'ts" of our lives; the Child represents spontaneous emotion and behavior; both Parent and Child must be governed by the Adult, the part of us that makes decisions based upon the objective facts. Coming at others from any one of these postures has predictable effects. We can often discover reasons for the disappointing responses we get from others by analyzing the particular posture from which we are approaching them. Literally thousands of people have found this book helpful in pursuing more positive feelings about themselves and relationships to others.

## Self-development

Most people agree that taking responsibility for ourselves and being honest in our view of reality is difficult. In *The Road Less Traveled*, psychiatrist M. Scott Peck integrates traditional spiritual and psychological insights regarding our performance of these tasks to give life its meaning and give us our mental health, or as Peck calls it, spiritual growth.[46] Life is composed of difficulties and suffering; this is common to us all. But the process of choosing to grow out of our difficulties sometimes requires choosing to suffer—the choice of a life of discipline. Discipline is motivated by love for ourselves and for others. Love is not easy and must consciously be chosen. Hence, we are called to take a hard look at our choices. Likewise, it is important that we examine how we view our world. Peck calls the view we hold of the world our religion, and understanding our religion or world view stimulates growth. Additionally, every organism that grows needs something outside of it helping it along. Peck calls this grace, the evidence of God—or the Force—if you will. It is a serendipitous power expressing itself through us by superseding our human abilities and wills and intervening on our behalf. Grace is our encourager; our own laziness is our evil. Simply stated, Peck suggests that neurosis is the proof of our laziness as we avoid suffering, discipline, love, and awareness. And mental difficulties are the indicator that this path is indeed wrong.

## ENDNOTES

1. Alvin Toffler, *Future Shock* (New York: Random House, 1970), 340–41.

2. Richard J. Riordan and Marilyn S. Beggs, "Counselors and Self-Help Groups," *Journal of Counseling and Development* 65 (1987): 427–29.

3. Jean Nidetch, *The Story of Weight Watchers* (New York: New American Library, 1972).

4. *St. Elizabeth's Reporter,* St. Elizabeth Hospital, Washington, D. C. (Summer, 1972), 2.

5. J. Norris, "World Dialogue on Alcohol and Drug Dependence," in *Alcoholics Anonymous,* ed. E. D. Whitney ( Boston: Beacon Press, 1970).

6. Clara C. Park and Leon N. Shapiro, *You Are Not Alone: Understanding and Dealing with Mental Illness* (Boston: Little Brown, 1979).

7. H. Grosz, Recovery, Inc., *Survey, Second Report* (Chicago, Inc., 1973).

8. Abraham A. Low, *Mental Health Through Will Training,* reprint of 1950 ed. (Boston: Willet, 1984).

9. *Recovery, Inc.: What It Is and How It Developed* (Chicago, Recovery, Inc., 1973).

10. *Some Principles of Emotions Anonymous* (St. Paul, Minnesota: Emotions Anonymous, 1983).

11. William Glasser, *Reality Therapy: A New Approach to Psychiatry* (New York: Harper Collins, 1975).

12. Rudolph Dreikurs, *Children: The Challenge* (New York: Dutton, 1991).

13. A. H. Katz and R. S. Bender, "Self-Help and Mutual Aid: An Emerging Social Movement?," *American Review of Sociology* 7 (1981): 129–155.

14. Richard J. Riordan and Marilyn S. Beggs, "Some Critical Differences Between Self-Help Groups and Therapy Groups," *Journal for Specialists in Group Work* 3, no. 1 (1988): 24–29.

15. F. Fiedler, "The Concept of an Ideal Therapeutic Relationship," *Journal of Consulting Psychology* 14 (1950): 239–45.

16. M. Lieberman, I. Yalom, and M. Miles, "Encounter: The Leader Makes the Difference," *Psychology Today* (March 1973): 70–76.

17. D. Truax and Robert Carkuff, *Towards Effective Counseling and Psychotherapy* (Chicago: Aldine, 1967).

18. H. Freed, K. Borus, J. Gonzales, J. Grant, O. Lightfoot, and V. Uribe, "Community Mental Health — Second-Class Citizen?," *Mental Health* 56 (Summer 1972).

19. S. Adams and M. Orgel, *Through the Mental Health Maze: A Consumer's Guide to Finding a Psychotherapist* (Washington, D.C.: Health Research Group, 1975).

20. Mario Puzo, *The Godfather* (New York: Putnam, 1969).

21. Albert Z. Carr, *Business As a Game* (New York: New American Library, 1969).

22. John Narcisco and David Burkett, *Declare Yourself: Discovering the Me in Relationships* (Englewood Cliffs, New Jersey: Prentice-Hall, 1975).

23. George Bach and Peter Wyden, *The Intimate Enemy: How To Fight Fair in Love and Marriage* (New York: Avon, 1976).

24. William J. Lederer and Don D. Jackson, *The Mirages of Marriage* (New York: W. W. Norton, 1968).

25. Mel Kranzler, *Creative Divorce* (New York: New American Library, 1974).

26. Fred Belliveau and Lin Richter, *Understanding Human Sexual Inadequacy* (Boston: Little Brown, 1970).

27. Boston Women's Health Collective, *The New Our Bodies, Ourselves: The Book by and for Women*, rev. ed. (New York: Simon and Schuster, 1985).

28. Sol Gordon, *The Sexual Adolescent: Communication with Teenagers about Sex* (North Scituate, Massachusetts: Duxbury Press, 1973).

29. James McCary, *A Complete Sex Education for Parents, Teenagers, and Young Adults* (New York: Van Nostrand Rheinhold, 1973).

30. Gerald R. Patterson, *Living with Children: New Methods for Parents and Teachers*, rev. ed. (Champaign, Illinois: Research Press, 1976).

31. Richard N. Bolles, *What Color Is Your Parachute? A Practical Manual for Job-Hunters and Career Changers* (Berkeley, California: Ten Speed Press, 1992).

32. John Holland, *Making Vocational Choices: A Theory of Careers* (Englewood Cliffs, New Jersey: Prentice-Hall, 1973).

33. Hans Selye, *The Stress of Life* (New York: McGraw Hill, 1956).

34. Hans Selye, *Stress Without Distress* (New York: New American Library, 1974).

35. Herbert Benson, *The Relaxation Response* (New York: Morrow, 1975).

36. Herbert Benson, *Beyond the Relaxation Response* (New York: Berkley Books, 1985).

37. Robert E. Alberti and Michael L. Emmons, *Your Perfect Right: A Guide to Assertive Living,* 6th ed. (San Luis Obispo, California: Impact Publications, 1990).

38. Jan D. Kelley and Barbara J. Winship, *I Am Worth It* (Chicago: Nelson Hall, 1979).

39. Arnold Lazarus and Allen Fay, *I Can If I Want To* (New York: Warner, 1988).

40. Manual J. Smith, *When I Say No, I Feel Guilty* (New York: Bantam, 1985).

41. Andrew Salter, *Conditioned Reflex Therapy* (New York: Creative Age Press, 1949).

42. Victor Frankl, *Man's Search for Meaning,* 3rd ed. (New York: Touchstone Books, 1984).

43. Huston Smith, *The Religions of Man* (New York: Harper-Collins, 1989).

44. Albert Ellis and Robert A. Harper, *The New Guide to Rational Living* (North Hollywood, California: Wilshire, 1976).

45. Thomas A. Harris, *I'm OK—You're OK: A Practical Guide to Transactional Analysis* (New York: Avon, 1976).

46. M. Scott Peck, *The Road Less Traveled* (New York: Simon and Schuster, 1985).

# EPILOGUE

Stress like change is an integral part of life. We will be totally free of stress only one time, and we are not looking forward to that option. As long as we are alive we must contend with stress. The goal, then, is the *management* of stress rather than its elimination. If Selye is correct in assuming that each of us has a limited and unrenewable amount of adaptation energy with which to deal with stressors, then learning to cope economically with them becomes literally a matter of life and death. This volume was written to assist readers to better understand the nature of stress, its sources, and to provide strategies for efficiently coping with it.

Much of this volume is concerned with creating an awareness of the consequences of stress on one's performance, one's relationships, and one's health. Stress in small doses is a tonic, adding energy and zest to life. Stress in large doses, however, is a killer! Chronic, unrelenting stress lowers immune efficiency, is responsible for a kind of chronic fatigue syndrome, robs us of the joy of life, ruptures our relationships with others, dulls our thinking capacity, and impairs our performance.

We have shown that we can prevent much stress by adopting wiser lifestyles — adjusting demands to a range of stimulation we find optimal for ourselves; pacing our efforts so that we function in a more centered, present mode; pursuing high-level wellness; and making wise choices, particularly of mates and vocations.

We have suggested effective ways of combating stress once we confront it. The key to successful combat is mind control—virtually all of our stress comes from our thinking. The body doesn't know the difference between fact and fantasy, and each time we entertain thoughts of frustration, failure, loss, or doom, the body gears up stressfully. Stress is not reality; it is our response to reality. "Out there" are merely persons, situations, and events. Whether these become stressful to us depends on the way we think about them. Stress results from a perception—the perception that our coping resources are not adequate to handle demands having serious consequences. We must persistently monitor and guide our thoughts to empower ourselves. Typically, we undercut our resources with pejorative self-references. We must recognize and appreciate the control we have over our situation.

A sense of control is critical in dealing with stressful situations. Body systems involved in dealing with stressors that we believe we can control are grossly different from those triggered by stressors we believe to be uncontrollable. Demands handled with a sense of control merely energize us; demands handled from a defensive, emotional crouch weaken and ultimately destroy us. Knowing this, we have repeatedly urged readers to empower themselves by doing the *unnatural* thing—that is, focusing on personal assets rather than on personal liabilities.

We further encouraged readers to learn to relax. A few minutes of healing silence will cool down an overly heated human machine. Meditation, deep muscle relaxation, prescribed breathing, listening to beautiful music, and taking quiet walks all serve as decompression chambers for escaping stressful mind sets. Our lives are pushy and noisy—we constantly push ourselves to do more, and we seem addicted to noise. Taking time out to be quiet and alone (not lonely) often works miracles of recuperation. We have emphasized also the enormous value of regular exercise as a means of de-stressing. A brisk walk or run will often burn up stress hormones and introduce a serene, restful state of consciousness.

Our experience as therapists has made us aware of how difficult it is to cause changes in the lifestyles of others. Self-change is too complicated to inspire in others if the inclination is not already there. While we are able to share with our readers beautiful stratagems for changing self-defeating habits, we do not know how to get others to use these stratagems with enough commitment to allow them to work. Our ignorance in this regard causes us to take comfort in Will Rogers' statement that "We're all ignorant . . . only on different subjects." We also comfort ourselves with the Zen aphorism, "When the pupil is ready, the teacher appears." We are convinced that certain approaches to change are more promising than others; consequently, we have reviewed the technology for change in order to strengthen the reader's efforts to change. We have tried to impress the reader with the vast reservoir of personal power that is his or hers for the using.

We have challenged the reader to give up favorite villains that may only serve as excuses for not investing the energy required to change. We attack beliefs that keep us from taking responsibility for our behavior and feelings: beliefs in powerful internal forces, past experiences, or environmental influences beyond our control that dwarf our efforts at self-determination. The reader was encouraged to use imagination to strengthen motivation, to engineer personal change through careful planning, and to make use of good books and good companions as assists to their resolve to change.

Success in self-change is sweet. To engineer our own change is exhilarating. Once we come to believe that we are capable of changing, the process itself is its own reward. Still, it is unquestionably the fate of humans to live and die with imperfection. Try as we may, there will always be things about ourselves that invite change. Indeed, the authors frequently cringe as they ponder their own imperfections while exhorting readers to move efficiently in correcting theirs. They fear the reader will expect that writers who profess some expertise in lighting the pathways to less stressful living will themselves be close to perfection. But life, perhaps, has no higher purpose than the unrelenting pilgrimage to become what we are capable of becoming. In this endeavor, fellow traveler, we wish you Godspeed.

# INDEX